Dear Pamela,

# 11 Vials

PETRA HOFFMANN

Although we have not met yet, I feel as though I know you.
Thankyou so much for becoming a part of my Incredible Journey!
To bright days ahead!
Love + Light, [signature]

First Edition – October 2011

**ISBN**
978-1-77067-898-9 (Hardcover)
978-1-77067-899-6 (Paperback)
978-1-77067-900-9 (eBook)



This is a work of non-fiction, and is about the author's own life. The names of the parties and characters have been changed to protect the innocent.

Published by:

FriesenPress
Suite 300 – 852 Fort Street
Victoria, BC, Canada V8W 1H8

www.friesenpress.com

Distributed to the trade by The Ingram Book Company

# Table of Contents

# Dedications

*I dedicate this book to three very special persons.*

*The first dedication goes out with all of my thanks and gratitude to:*

*Gordon Everett Koett – may you forever rest in peace my friend.*

*I thank you Gord, for seeing my potential, teaching me to love myself, and ultimately saving my life.*

*The second dedication goes out to my daughter with all of my heart and all of my soul, to:*

*Kayla Deanna Koett – I love you to infinity and beyond my baby dolly!*

*Thank you for coming into my life, loving me unconditionally and giving me reason to live.*

*The third dedication goes out to the love of my life:*

*Eli M. Telo – thank you for believing in me, taking care of me when I needed you to, and for being the driving force behind my "finishing something" for the first time in my life.*

*A final huge thanks goes out to my special "Angels on Earth"*

*You know who you are!*

Do you know that you DON'T have it?

- 500 million people worldwide are currently infected with Hepatitis B or C
- This is over 12 times the number infected with HIV/AIDS
- Between them, hepatitis B and C kill 1.5 million people a year
- One in every three people on the planet has been exposed to either or both viruses
- Most of the 500 million infected do not know it

**PANDEMIC!** 1 in 12 people globally has Hepatitis C, as stated in a 1998 Press Release by the World Health Organization!

# Prelude

Does it matter if you don't know whether to start at the beginning or the end? Does it really matter how the story is told, just so long as it is told? There are friends and family who will disagree with some of what I am going to share with you here. I remember things my way, in my reality. I realize as I write this and tell my story, that others will recall the same events differently. All I do know, is that for many years now, I have had a voice in my head telling me to write a book! My life has rarely ever been boring, and I have a lot of stories to tell. What I don't know for sure, is whether anyone really gives a damn about my life. I suppose that I won't know unless I try, right? I would like to think that perhaps through my sharing my world, I may help others understand themselves better.

I keep thinking lately, that if the whole world does go up in flames, so to speak, then I would like to be left with a lot of pens and paper. That way I may be able to keep writing. The world is a volatile place today, and no one really knows what will transpire next. I keep thinking, that as I look forward at whatever scene stands before me, no matter what room I may be in...that the entire scenario could change at any moment. I envision it like going through a worm hole, strategically placed, and finding myself in another dimension.

You know what? I'm open. Everything these days makes sense, and paradoxically nothing makes sense. I asked the almighty Universe today to tell me what my true vocation is. What am I supposed to do now? Is it Real Estate or something else, like this book? Well, I believe that I am now committed to this project. Maybe, just maybe, you are at this very moment looking through the looking glass, at the very moment in time, that my forté reveals itself to me. I also know inside myself that I want to help other people. By that, I think that would be mentally speaking...and to get the word out. Yes, the world at this time is facing unlimited avenues of destruction. Everything is striking us at once. I believe that we need to get the word out, and I would be willing, if the Universe wished it, to try to help or educate others. I would like to show them how to step over to the side of love and kindness, and a belief system so strong, that I believe possibly, just maybe, we will get the opportunity to take some sort of a quantum leap. The scenarios are limitless. It certainly is an exciting time to be here, the leaps in technology, and technology we, as humankind may only ever be able to imagine. That's the truth, right there, we have more power than we will ever know, or maybe ever even realize.

I hope by now that most of you have a sense of the whole (all of us) being connected. I feel really grateful right now. Of all the mundane computer things I do, this is by far the most enjoyable. I actually like this writing so much, that it really doesn't seem like work. Everything else I do does. I don't know quite how to explain this, because I've reached an extreme level of this unique problem I seem to have. I am physically really lazy. I hate exercise more than anyone I have ever met in my life, and I am not exaggerating. Even if nobody ever wants to read this book, I believe now that it will help me to get all these stories out. My loved ones are sick of hearing them over and over again. They will finally be released, for the last time, so that I can concentrate more on the "Now." Which brings me to which...the book that changed me as the Being I once was, is titled "*The Power of Now*", by Eckart Tolle.

I began reading book after self-help book since the Power of Now, and they all seem to point to one thing. Stay in the Now and when it all becomes too much to handle, sit still and do nothing. The hardest obstacle for me at this particular point in time is to try not to worry about the bills I cannot pay. I need to learn to trust that if I don't let it eat me up inside, that the Universe will provide. I also tell myself now, that if I simply cannot jump a certain hurtle, then I will just go around it, and in turn be on a new adventure. I have never in my life encountered so many obstacles as I have in the last few years.

# Chapter 1 - The Proverbial Childhood

Alright, so now, let's attempt to start at the beginning of my story. Allow me to begin simply, by telling you where I was born. It was a tiny little town called Iserlohn, once more in Germany. My brother, who is seven years my junior, was literally made in Germany and born in Canada. We came to Vancouver, British Columbia, Canada in 1967 when I was almost seven years old, and half way through grade one. We travelled here together with my aunt and uncle, who were also pregnant with my cousin, both boys having been conceived in Germany. My parents, both being full blooded Germans came here with $2,000 dollars in dad's pocket and a dream. My memories in years that would lie ahead, of Germany, came back to me in nightmares. My fondest memories are however, of Italy, where we used to go on vacation about twice a year. I remember even the little VW Bug and the tent, and rubber dinghy. I believe in my heart, that it was because of the ocean that I loved Italy so very much. I live near the coast now, and cannot imagine ever living anywhere without the ocean. It is the only place in the whole wide world where I find my inner peace. I find it every single time that I go out there, without fail, no matter what is going on in my life.

I seriously was not going to make this book about my parents and my childhood, but that has proven to be impossible, and I have since changed my mind. My childhood moulded me into who I am today, and although I truly believed that I had dealt with all my issues, I now realize that I was completely wrong. You see, the way we grow up and were raised is mostly thought of by us as "normal." That is because we know no other way than the way we are taught, until we grow older and wiser. The way I remember my childhood is that when we were still living in Germany, I was the centre of my parents' attention. They doted on me when I was little. Mom dressed me up in designer clothes...you know, the cute little dresses, with the matching coat, shoes, and of course the hat to match? I still do, to this day, love hats.

My mom and dad both worked a lot, and I was left in a preschool run by nuns. I loved it there, and as I recall I was treated really well. At the age of five however, I started school. There is no kindergarten in Germany, they start you right off in grade one. I think we started at 8am and went to school until 1pm in the afternoon. They sent you home though, with about four or five hours worth of homework right from the very first day. Talk about going from 0-90! Well, after school, I had to attend this other daycare service, which was right across the street from school. This part of my life came back to me in nightmares many years later. I realize now that I had learned how to block out bad experiences from a very young age. I was severely mistreated in this daycare, by the other kids, and the staff turned a blind eye, and told me not to be a cry baby. I hated every single second of it. Thank Gosh that we moved to Canada before the year was even out.

Life, as I knew it, changed first, of course when we flew to Canada, and shortly thereafter, when my little brother was born. Don't get me wrong, I loved my little brother, but did I have to become a part of the wallpaper that quickly and efficiently? My brother soon became my mom and dad's everything, and from then on, I felt as though I became their slave. Listen, I didn't choose to have a kid, they did. So why did he become my responsibility? Whenever he fussed, my mom would make me take him out for a walk. It was not long before I became extremely resentful. Not only was I overlooked now, but who was the brat's mother? How come I had to do everything? My friends soon got tired of walking Petra's brother, so now they left me out of their games, and would go off without me all the time.

Well, Petra's little brother soon grew. I had to stay home and babysit him, rather than go out and play. Never, ever, was I allowed to have friends come to my house, to play with me either. They might mess up the house, ask for food, water or something, you know? It is sad to think about it now. There was only one exception. I was allowed to invite three friends, and three friends only, to have over for my sixteenth birthday party. We had to stay outside as they were not allowed in. Wow...thank Gosh my parents thought the Sweet Sixteen milestone was so special! Anyway, as my brother grew, it got even worse. I would try to escape, because here's the other thing...I was forbidden to play in the house. Whenever possible, my mom would make us go outside to play, so we didn't mess up the house. If and when we were indoors, we would be sent to our rooms.

When first moving to Canada, I was a bit of a tomboy, and liked to play with the boys and climb trees and such. The problem was I only had the designer dresses we had brought from Germany.

Other than my "lederhosen" I did not even own any pants. Well... that didn't sit well with my mom, and I always got in trouble when I came home and my clothes were dirty. I actually ended up getting spankings over it. My mom was the one who used to cuff me across the head, but I do not remember her ever really hitting me, like my dad did. He would just hit me wherever he could. I got hit in the head so many times, it is a wonder I don't have brain damage. Normally, though, he would go straight for the wooden spoons, and then make me bend over while he broke them on my ass, and my back. I often had welts and bruises there. Finally, finally, and believe me it was not easy, I talked my mom into buying me my first pair of jeans. I totally remember them; they were GWG Scrubbies, which we bought at Army and Navy. It was one of the most winning moments of my childhood existence, it had been far from easy to convince her to let me wear pants, and allow me to get them dirty. I actually succeeded, and that, my friends, was not something they let me do often. Normally I would not have been allowed to discuss the topic. I was never allowed to voice my opinions or express any emotions. Children were to be seen, not heard.

Throughout my childhood, what I remember most is they gave me shit for everything I did or didn't do. They were always putting me down. Never do I remember any show of affection from my parents towards me. They never bent down to hug or kiss me, or even tell me that they loved me. I never recall them telling me they were proud of me. That's why it was such a big deal the first time I ever heard those words come from my father's mouth. It was the day that I took my Real Estate exam the first time. I was so sure that I had passed the test. I called my dad from the first payphone I saw, to tell him. He was my very first call, and it was the first time I had heard him say that he was proud. It literally brought me to tears on the phone. I will never forget the feeling of elation when he said those words to me. It validated my entire existence in that moment. That's how much I suppose I must have craved some sort of affirmation. I think it was only because I was now following in his footsteps somewhat, because he is a home contractor.

As my little brother got a bit older, my mom would send him out with me, and when my friends wanted to go and play somewhere, I would have to drag him along. I hated it, and so did my friends. Thinking back on it now, it must not have made him feel so great either. There was this one time, when I had gone outside to play, and I really did not want to come in for dinner, and my mom had already called me in a few times. I pretended not to hear her, and soon found out, that that was a most terrible mistake on my part. Just for that, and nothing else, (although to this day, I have never admitted to having heard her calling me in the first place) she and dad grounded me for the whole of the summer holidays that year. Not only was I grounded and not allowed to leave the backyard, but they put me to work. It took all summer, but I had to paint their fuckin' white picket fence that scorching hot year, not to mention everything else they needed to get done. I hated them! And the worst part was also, that I was never allowed to vent my anger. I was not allowed to cry, I was not allowed to scream, I could not show any of my real feelings, ever! I was too scared, the fear had been too deeply ingrained. I worked hard at first, I thought maybe they would feel sorry for me and let me off my grounding, but that day never came. At that age (about 8 or 9 at the time), an entire summer might as well be a lifetime. This is what jail might feel like, only in jail you would have people to talk to. I had nobody, except once in a long while this girl, who had just moved in next door, would come outside and shyly communicate with me through the white picket fence. Gosh, how I grew to hate that fence! She was East Indian though, and knew no English, so communication was stilted to say the least. I felt sorry for her, because when summer was over, and I was again allowed out, I ended up leaving her all alone, and I felt bad about that.

A couple of years afterwards, we moved to Tsawwassen (a neighbouring suburb, named by Natives as "The Home of the Sungod.") at the age of 12. There, life for me became worse yet. First off, the kids were so different, and now, I was not allowed out at all anymore, or so it seemed. I was older, and capable of doing way more work, I suppose. The first thing I recall is the giant mountains of soil, which my dad had hauled into the front of the yard, up by the road, beside the driveway. It became my job for the next couple of months or so, to shovel that crap into an old beat up, rickety green wheelbarrow, with spindly little wheels that were about to break. It was the stupidest little wheelbarrow I had ever seen, nothing like the ones that normal people would buy. But, he was too cheap to fork out any money to buy a stronger one. If the job was difficult, he could keep me home longer. So, I had to shovel, get it first to the backyard, where we began, and then to the front yard, dump it, and spread it with a rake. It was intensely difficult work for me, for I was always a skinny, frail girl. I do not recall how many months it took me to complete this task, but it seemed like forever.

The yard in question was about a half acre in size, not a small yard to maintain. Dad then put all the gardens, and hedges in, and planted seed, with me by his side of course. He always kept me by his side whenever he had any work to do in the yard, or in the garage. He hated to do tasks on his own I suppose. My father has never done well alone, not for a single day. He might have to look in the mirror, should that ever happen. He used to make me hold the trouble light when there was a hook on the wall right behind me, just to keep me there. Not only to be by his side, but to keep me home, and away from boys. After the gardens were complete, guess who had to maintain everything? He mowed the grass, and rather than use a catcher, he made me rake it. I had to rake the leaves about twice a week in the fall as well. I had to keep the weeds out of all the gardens. I had to...ok, here was the schedule, as I recall it, actually. Friday afternoons, after school, while all my friends were elsewhere, I was cleaning the entire downstairs of our two story five bedroom home. That, of course, was after I had also been my dad's aid to build the basement. Oh, the temper tantrums I remember him having, as he attempted to lift the gyp-rock to the ceiling with the help of a frail wisp of a twelve year old girl. I was so skinny when I was a child, by the way, that after I moved from Vancouver, I was made fun of in school every single bingle day. Each day was another day of being bullied, in my life in good old sunny Tsawwassen. And the tantrums he used to have under his car and in his garage! On Saturdays I had to wash the car and shimmy it dry. I also had to wash the underside of the car, and once a month I had to wax shine the car. Not just the car, but also that big green Chevy work van he used to have. Every Saturday, he would then come and inspect it. If there were any streaks left on the car, or water drops, I would have to do it over. He even checked the underneath, and I would hold my breath, in case he saw any mud left there. The raking, and weeding, and general yard maintenance, and the driveways, walkways, etc., I was to do after school during the week. No wonder I never did my homework. I just had a flood of memories, and realize that I have never allowed myself to think about a lot of the details of my childhood. I remember vividly now, the days and nights, when he would be so stubborn, or he would be so mad at me, for whatever reason, and he would leave me out there in the cold darkness, working. My hands would be almost frost bitten sometimes, and then I had to pick up the pace to keep myself warm. It was like torture, pure torture, so many days and nights. My fingers, thumbs, and feet would often be covered in blisters that would bleed.

My father did whatever he could think of to keep me home. As I grew and especially when I reached my teenage years, there was nothing he wouldn't do to keep me at home and not out with my friends. I don't think he could stand the thought of me having any fun. What if I were to meet or spend time with a boy? He would not be able to endure it. Whatever he could do to prevent that, he would do. I realized that if I hurried through my chores so I could go out, he would just give me more chores. So I learned to take my time, and endure getting yelled at and threatened instead. When the chores ran dry, I would be made to work in the garage with my Papa. A favourite chore of his, when he had run out of everything else, was to get me to sort the nails from the screws. (THESE WERE IN 10 GALLON DRUMS, FOLKS!) Get this: when I had that accomplished (years worth of work), he would get me to "categorize" the nails and screws. Basically, here I was, tucked away with only dad and I in the garage. There I was demeaned and abused wholeheartedly by my father. I realize in trying to tell the story that I have blocked out the most of it, because it is extremely hazy to me. I find myself wondering, now, also, why it is that my mother never did come and check on me in that damned garage. I don't recall her, not even once, coming in to check on things. She must have heard the yelling and screaming. All I know is that if it were my daughter, I would go check once in a while, and wonder what they were up to for so long. Nope, not her though.

Now let me tell you about that night that scarred me for the rest of my life. It tainted sex quite badly for me. I was raised (it serves mention here) that sex is bad, dirty, and disgusting, and that you should never do it at all until you are married. So, here is the story about Jerry and me. Jerry is the boy whom I was totally in love with for five years throughout high school. So was every other girl in Tsawwassen! And Jerry Cook took advantage of that, and yes, he was the school slut! One evening, I arrived at home after the pool hall, and my mom and dad were still out. I took this opportunity to take our dog for a walk around the block. Yes, yes, in hopes of seeing Jerry. Well, turns out I did, how lucky was I? Didn't take us long, we ended up necking, (it was a beautiful, sultry, summer night) behind the hedges in his front yard. One thing led to another. Jerry had convinced me to tie the dog up to the car under the carport. What happened next, was one of my most incredible experiences. I think it was the first time I felt that "horny" feeling. After a lot of heavy petting and touching, my pants came down, and for the first time in my young life, I knew I was ready. I was going to let him have my virginity, and I was completely in the moment and fully conscious. Jerry was just about to enter, and I mean, just about to enter, (like in right then and there) and who comes around the fucking corner of the hedge? Who do I see looming right above me? My friggin' Papa! Fear gripped me so intensely, that it felt as though someone was squeezing my heart. I have never in my entire life been so scared, so completely terrified! He pulled Jerry off of me, and with his pants around his ankles, Jerry was unable to fight back. My dad hit and kicked the crap out of him. I could only watch in horror, as thoughts raced through my mind that he might kill him, or hurt him really badly.

Then he left Jerry lying on the lawn in a heap and started towards me. I had obviously been sitting there immobilized in fear, because I had made no move to pull up my pants. The next thing I knew he was lifting me up off the grass, and I remember, (oh so vividly), pissing myself right then and there. Have you ever been so scared you have actually pissed yourself? What a horrible feeling. Then, before I knew it, I found myself airborne, and my glasses went flying. I saw Jerry pick himself up and stagger to the house, before I was somehow whisked away. The rest is a blur, I recall my mom's presence there, but have no idea where she was while all of this was happening. I remember her there, only because I heard both their voices as though in a dream, just before I had seen my Papa looming over me.

I wish that I had somehow been able to believe that it would be over, but alas, that's why the blur. The next thing I remember is being thrown backwards onto our living room couch, and Papa was spitting in my face, calling me a whore and a slut. The next words out of his mouth stand out so vividly, for he used the same threat for many more years to come. He screamed at me that he could hardly wait until I had kids, so that he could tell them what I had done, and what a tramp their mother is. I think my Mama was in the living room with us then, but again, I am not sure.

The next thing I recall was being pulled off the couch, thrown to the floor, and kicked over to the top of the staircase. He then picked up a spike heeled shoe, and tried to smash my head with it. As I covered my head he threw me down the stairs, or I may have fallen, I am not quite sure. Landing at the bottom, I looked up into his raging eyes. I knew then that if I did not get up and run, I would be dead. I ran to my right, into the basement and almost made it to the door. I had my hand on the doorknob, but it was too late, and I felt him right behind me. I was so close, but to no avail. The next thing I knew, he threw me in the corner behind the door by my hair, and his big hands went around my throat. He was literally choking me out. I thought he was going to kill me, really and truly. It is the only time my Papa ever laid a hand on me, (and there were many) that I heard my Mama intervene. She was right behind him, and tried to pull him off of me. I think I heard her say, in German, "that is enough, stop it, stop it, that is enough." Thank Gosh he listened, she somehow had gotten through to him, without getting hurt herself. I assume that was why she never stepped in before. I think she was scared too.

I do not recall my dad ever hitting my mom, but my brother told me that he had witnessed him try. He stepped between them once. My mom told me that he had hit her when they were still dating before they got married. She threatened that if he ever laid a hand on her again, she would pick up a frying pan or something, and do some serious damage. From the way I understand it, he never laid a hand on her again.

After that night, my parents kept me home from school for a week. Poor Jerry had to go back with not one but two, black eyes. The kids had a hay day with him. My glasses were never to be seen again. Jerry said he looked for them, and I certainly couldn't go back there to look (what must the neighbours have thought, and why did no one jump in?) My parents wouldn't buy me new glasses and so I had to go to school blind as a bat until I could save up enough money to buy them myself. I began work from the time I was sixteen years old.

One day when we were all at my aunt and uncle's Silver Wedding anniversary, years after I had moved out, I began to talk about my childhood. We were sitting in the living room, and had all had more than a couple of drinks. I had just heard one more time, something that I have heard so many times over the years. A couple that were also there, told me that they had known my mom and dad for more than ten years. "They knew they had a son, but they didn't know they had a daughter." "Strange," I thought, "since this woman is my aunt's best friend, also?" I would hear this same sentence from many more people, whom I was to meet in life. So, in front of the family and a few close friends, I asked my father why he had always been that overprotective of me as a child. He admitted to me, and everybody else that day, that if he could have kept me in a glass case in the living room, he would have done exactly that. "And," he added, "I have always been more jealous of you, than I have ever been of my wife." I shot a quick look at my mom and saw the pain in her eyes, for that was the most honest thing he had ever said. Suddenly it all made some semblance of sense to me. He did not ever want me to meet a boy and fall in love, and be taken away from him. That was why he kept me home working.

I wonder if he ever really knew how hard he truly was on me. Another chore I forgot to tell you about was that once a week, I had to shine and polish all of his shoes. His work boots were more difficult as they had to be cleaned, dried, and treated with special oils and goops. He used to make me give me back massages once or twice a week also, when he came home from work. Sometimes he paid me a quarter for this service. Then, he'd do strange things, such as pay me to eat banana peppers, while he watched my pain with great amusement. He has also offered to pay me to touch jelly fish, when we were out boating. He'd tell me they were harmless, and that their sting (which really wouldn't hurt at all) was medicinal. He used to tell me that Indians walked purposely through poison ivy, for medicinal purposes, and that I should do the same. When I refused he would offer to pay me to do it.

One day, I will never forget, was when he came home from work and offered me his special treat that mom used to make in his lunch. She used to peel and section oranges, and then douse them with tons of sugar, and they were his favourite. I mean, he would never offer them to his kids, not ever before. That day though, he magnanimously, offered them to me, saying he had been too full to finish his lunch. I felt so damn special that afternoon, and wondered what I had done right to deserve such a treat! I happily opened the see through "Dell jam" container (I remember it so vividly, as though it were only yesterday). With eyes as big as saucers, I peered into the top. There was the perfect slice, with a ton of sugar, right there on top! He watched every move in rapt silence. I brought the succulent piece to my mouth and bit into it, closing my eyes in anticipation of the huge burst of juice and sugar on my tongue. The next thing I knew, I was gagging and spewing, and felt my face turn beet red. I knew not to make a mess, or my mom would be mad, as I ran to the bathroom, and puked. My dad followed me all the way laughing like it was the funniest thing he had ever seen. I mean there were tears in his eyes, from laughing so hard. I looked to my mom to help me, but she only looked on in total sympathy. I realize now, as I sit and write this, that she never ever, ever, stuck up for me. Never would she say a word, other than, "That wasn't very nice, Evan," or something to that effect. If she did say anything there would, of course, be a big giant, full blown fight. You see, what had happened was that, my mom had mixed up the sugar and the salt. Of course, I had chosen the piece with the most "sugar."

Every single day that I can remember of my childhood, my parents fought. They fought all the time, and as we grew older it seemed to get even worse. Every day they argued about "grocery money." At dinner time, we all had to sit at one table, because that was the law. No one ever broke that rule no matter what. At dinner we were to be together, as a family. Wow, the dinners. Let me try to even describe the suppers at the Hoffmann table, day in, and day out. There was a fight at the dinner table most every night. Usually, it would start off quietly. Something would be said that was of course, wrong, and then they would start bickering again, the incessant bickering. It was all we knew. We called my dad the "garbage eater." I always had to eat whatever was put on my plate. The only thing I was allowed to do, was cut the fat off my meat. It literally made me vomit. I cannot swallow fat, to this day. Well, dad would eat all of our fat. And dad would also eat anything left over on anybody's plate, no matter how big or small, because he didn't want to waste it. Sometimes, I thought he might explode.

He didn't care, he forced it down because "there were starving people in the world."

Notice how I have barely mentioned my mom? Well...my mom, thought by others to be "cold as a cucumber," can be just that. It just never occurred to me until I began this book, that my mom never did defend me. I did not feel any warmth or love exude from her throughout my childhood. I felt no emotion from her towards me, other than loathing and dislike somehow. I didn't realize all that then, of course. As I said before, I did not know any different. For me it was normal behaviour. I remember feeling as if she liked me every now and then, but only small glimpses. My Mama was totally different with my younger brother though. She absolutely loved him. He could do no wrong in her eyes. My mom to this day, and I have to say, (and I believe it to be even worse now), detaches herself from life as we know it. She lives in her own bubble, and has a way of simply not acknowledging anything she can't accept, or do anything about. Being a mother myself, I can't understand how anyone could let another person treat their own flesh and blood so badly. I think she only cared about what the neighbours would think. We were disciplined beyond normal measures.

I used to be "daddy's little girl" when I was little, when we were still in Germany, before my brother was born. For most of my life I had blocked this out, but having had a few dreams about it, I asked my mom for more details. She filled in the blanks, and it all came rushing back to me. Every Sunday, my dad would take me for a walk in the woods near our apartment. He used to dote on me, and spoil me like crazy back in those days. I was raised in an "open marriage" partnership, but the rules I believe were broken, even back then. I recall one sunny Sunday when my dad took me out for our weekly walk. I did not ever really question why (for I was only four or five at the time), he would always leave me in the same spot, and tell me not to move. Then he would go off alone down another path, and reappear a while later. I had no concept then of how much time he would be gone, but I think it varied.

Well, one day curiosity set in, and although I was really scared, and I knew that I would be in so much trouble if I left my spot, I decided to follow him. It was as though I were in a trance. It was a short distance, before we came upon a little clearing and there was a woman. She was really pretty, and I think she had long dark hair. She was a stranger to me, but the next thing I knew, my Papa was kissing this stranger. I could not grasp this at all, and had blocked it out until a few years ago, when it came back to me. It was after something my Mama had said about my dad cheating on her, with his best friend's wife. I described to her the woman in my hazy memories, and she confirmed that that was her. Dad used to meet her in the woods, and mom had found out about it back then.

My parents told me about their "open marriage" when I was approximately twelve years old, and I did not have a clue what that even meant then. I think that title was invented after his many indiscretions. I don't know how to explain it to you so you can comprehend it, because it is so, so unclear to me, yet at the same time crystal clear. I have always told myself that I am so lucky because at least I was not sexually abused like so many people I know today. People have a way of opening themselves up to me as though I am a magnet to their tales. They seem to sense that they can trust me with their deepest darkest secrets, and they have told me things that I can never repeat. The thing of it is that you have to know me well enough to swear me to secrecy and if you forget, I may share the info with others. I think I would be a pretty good counsellor actually. It's the thought of more schooling that sucks. I realize now that although there was no actual sexual abuse there certainly WAS physical and most definitely, a ton of mental abuse. No wonder I put up with it from my first boyfriend, which you will hear all about soon enough.

My first years of school in East Vancouver were my best years of school. Well, the beginning was a bit rough with the language barrier. I also was a scrawny little runt, and everyone picked on me and beat me up a lot. I came home bloody almost everyday for a while. My mom finally answered the front door one day, and told me in no uncertain terms, that she was not going to feel sorry for me anymore, and that I have to hit back from now on. She added, "but don't you ever let me catch you hitting first, or I will hit you myself." Well, I heard her, and in no time at all, I became one of the biggest scrappers in school. I would provoke the fights when I didn't like somebody, but I never hit first. I think I got out most of my frustration that way, for the next few years.

My two best friends who were really pretty and we became the most popular girls in that school. It was so great. I remember it feeling just as in my imaginings of celebrity status, you know what I mean? Things were going really well. I had my first real crush on the hottest guy in school (Sarah and I, both would try to outdo each other in our love notes we'd sneak into his desk). Of course it was then, that my parents decided it was time to pull up roots, and we moved to a nearby suburb, a town called Tsawwassen. This transpired half way through grade six, when I was twelve years old. Over the years, many people have asked about the effects and culture shock I must have felt moving from Germany to Canada, but the real shock came when I moved to Tsawwassen. It was a rich town, full of stuck up snotty nosed brats, not at all like the "down to earth" tougher city kids. They were so mean to me. I did not fit in at all. They were like aliens to me. It was then that I became a geeky book worm. It was better than to try to be someone I was not.

In high school, and after I had finished my "torrid affair" with Jerry Cook, I fell "in love" with another guy that all the girls in school were in love with. Tim took full advantage of them all, inclusive of myself. I did not actually lose my virginity (to him), until I was almost 19 years old. There's a great story...and not a girl's dream of "that special night," that is for sure! I had already been kicked out of the house and it was my last year of school. I was at a huge party with my best friend, whose parents had taken me in. Nearing the end of the party, I was invited over to Tim's house. He had promised to make me a "bacon and tomato sandwich", and being gooned, I believed him. That night was horrid. You know it must be bad when you are that friggin' drunk and everything is still so awkward. It all just felt so wrong, and I never got the sandwich either. Instead I got to sneak out of his f...in bedroom window, hung over as a dog. He had shooed me out when his mom began nagging at his bedroom door at 6 o'clock in the freakin' morning. It was a long, cold walk home. Especially in torn nylons and high heels, really long.

Now, here's the part I love to tell. About twenty years later, a friend from school invited me to his cousin's wedding. I recall so clearly, waiting in our limo for the others to arrive. Tim was the first to arrive, only I did not recognize him at all. From being the most attractive guy in town, he was now almost completely bald and really ugly. It's funny how that happens to some people. I would not have believed it, had I not seen it with my own eyes.

That's kind of like what happened to me in reverse. Since I had become a geek in school (for my mother dressed me like one to boot), I was voted the female most changed at my ten year high school reunion. Guys that did not even know who I was before, were literally pushing one another aside to have their pictures taken with ME! It was one of the best feel good nights, I have ever endured. It was so great that the same group of witches, whom had spent so much energy making fun of me for all those years, sat in one corner all night judging everyone just as they had always done in school. At the end of the night a whole bunch of us went back to an after party at someone's house. A couple of different guys told me that the same girls had had a bet going on whether I was wearing any underwear or not. Sheesh...all they had to do was ask. I'd have shown them! lol

Although I did not graduate since I was one elective short, I was still invited to the grad dinner and dance. The dinner was at the Commodore Ball Room, one of my favourite venues in Vancouver. My parents were never there for any of my events anyway, but I still found myself wondering if they would not appear? I had wished for them to buy me some contact lenses for the occasion, but they were too cheap. My glasses were literally "coke bottle bottoms", and so, I attended blind. At that dinner (I later discovered) were some talent scouts. They were to pick one girl from Tsawwassen and one from a neighbouring town called Ladner, to compete in the "Miss Delta Pageant 1979." The rest of the contestants signed up themselves.

After the grad ceremonies, my phone started ringing...by now I had had several people tell me that they had been asking people about me that night. If you know me now, you would not be able to believe it, but I was really shy in high school. Of course I quietly told them "Thank you, but no, I do not want to participate." Well, they were very persistent and after the fifth call, I finally relented. As it turned out, it was one of the best experiences of my life. I overcame so many personal hurtles. I was in the newspapers, on local television, meeting, and trying to impress, and being interviewed by some very intimidating people to me. For example, at the pool party, we had to be challenged one on one, by a panel of five or six judges. That was really difficult for me. The night of the actual pageant, is a blur. I do not remember my impromptu speech at all, but I know that I said something about concerts and received a standing ovation. Miss Vancouver and Miss Surrey later sought me out to congratulate me, and tell me that they thought my speech was better than anyone else's. That felt pretty good.

I began, (and I just thought I would leap right in with this) drugs the first time when I was 16 years old. A friend of mine had a show horse, and I was asked by the kids that hung out at the barn, whether I smoked pot. I didn't want them to think I was a suck hole, so I told them that of course I did. Well, I'll let you guess the rest...doesn't take a rocket scientist. It was very soon after that happened that I started hanging out with this girl who lived alone with her father, and was a very dark and unhappy girl. Mona was a total "head." She smoked pot any chance she got, and her father gave her a really good allowance. She bought me a bong, for my sixteenth birthday, so I guess I was actually fifteen, when I first smoked pot. Although I have lost everything more than once in my life, the odd things remained sacred, and that bong is still with me today. It serves as a constant reminder of days I never wish to repeat, for of course, I have loaded it with other things as well. I still, to this day, smoke pot, but you will soon come to understand that that is (well it is to me) nothing. Apparently, I am wrong about that, but I can live with it. One day I may quit, who knows, but it isn't going to be today. To throw you back to the present with me, though, I actually did quit smoking cigarettes two years ago in October. I started when I was sixteen. My uncle was in the hospital, it was a Friday night, and he pretty much cut out twice that afternoon. All I could think was, "I do not want to die that way," and without further ado, I quit. I even went back to my brother's place that evening, and he and his girlfriend are complete chain smokers. I sat there all night with them, and I have never had another drag off a cigarette since...yet, (for being an addict and having fallen back more than once, I have learned to never say never).

Another experience that stands out in my mind now that happened to me while I was still in high school, was the time I ended up at a huge party in the neighbouring town, right on the river. I do not recall who I had gone there with, but found myself at daybreak having been left behind, with only a very few stragglers remaining. I remember talking to Mick Jergen on the front stoop of the house, while we shared a cigarette. He was a very charismatic, good looking guy that many girls had a crush on. His girlfriend for the most part of high school was a beautiful model. I mean, she was stunning. What transpired next, when we went back into the house to the living room, was completely unexpected. His two friends were sitting on the couch. Mick and I sat on the floor of the room, and the next thing I know, he had me pinned down on the ground, right in front of his buddies. He was on top of me, and actually tried to rape me right then and there. It was Shane, his best friend who I remember jumped up first, and then both boys pulled Mick off of me. Thank Gosh for small miracles. I had a feeling that this was not the first time they had been witness to this kind of abuse.

I later found out that Mick had raped at least five other girls at school. He lives in Tsawwassen to this day. I ran into him at the pub there about a year ago. He ended up on heroin and is now doing crack. He was completely tweaking when I saw him, and he proceeded to follow me everywhere. He even went so far as to tell me that he does not drink, as he kept picking up a pint of beer. "Total loser," I thought, as I told him to get lost, and that I could care whether he drank or not.

Remembering this story, brings back another memory of the New Years Eve party my parents had when I was also in high school. My friend, whom I had grown up with in East Vancouver and her mom, came over for the celebrations. My dad had bought us two girls a magnum of Baby Duck sparkling wine and when we ran out, he gave us some Apple Jack wine. This cheap wine was well known to be really potent. Needless to say, Kerry and I got hammered, and decided to go out to a party. So, we went and said "Good night," to our parents, then went back to my room and put pillows and stuff under the covers, so that they would think we were in there. The slut of a guy that I had always been "in love" with in school, the one my dad had beaten up earlier, was having a big party that night. We went over there to check it out, it was just around the block from my house. I was scared to stay too long and figured we should go check in at home. Unfortunately, we were caught by the cops. We were out after curfew, so he wanted to drive us home. I begged and pleaded that he drop us off at the church across the road from my house, "because my dad will kill me." The officer was pretty nice and complied. We checked in, and then snuck out again, and were rounded up by the same cop about half way around the block. Again, I begged for the church parking lot, and again he complied... until he caught us the third time, that is. The third time, we didn't have a chance. He took us straight to the door, and rang the bell. I was absolutely terrified! I will never forget my dad being called to the door. He was livid. He asked the officer if he too had a daughter, and when the cop replied, "No," my father shoved me hard into his arms and said, "Here, have this one." The police officer proceeded to tell him that since I was only sixteen, he had to take me back into the house. So, dad waited until the cop car had pulled out of the driveway, and dumb ass me had taken off my coat and boots, (for it was snowing heavily outside). He then grabbed me, opened the front door, and threw me barefoot out into the snow. I made it about two blocks before my girlfriend's mom pulled up beside me, and they took me back home with them to Richmond. I ended up there for about a week. The following Sunday, my parents came over to collect me. No apologies, it was entirely my fault.

When I was about eighteen, I started hanging out with a friend of a roommate's, who had moved downtown Vancouver. My "roommate" at the time was my best friend Mandy, whose parents were kind enough to take me in when I got kicked out for my last year of school. I will always be grateful to that family for what they did for me. Anyways, I ended up with Mandy's friends ex boyfriend, and didn't have the guts to tell her about it. I would tell my parents that I was going to her house and before long I was caught. She called my parents and ratted me out. I got kicked out of the house for the fifth and final time. After that, I moved home for about two months and then moved out again, and have never been back.

I guess it would have been the latter part of 1979 or the beginning of 1980, that I ended up (and I cannot remember how) at a bar in a neighbouring, much larger metropolis, called Surrey. Surrey has always had a bad rap of being the seediest part of Greater Vancouver. It is also the largest city (was a municipality then) in Canada, so in my opinion, of course it has more crime. I started seeing this guy, Roy, whom I met there, and was soon introduced to all his "party animal" friends. I was embarking on a new adventure, let me be telling you! He and I lasted about two months, and then he dumped me and moved on to someone else. It was a bit later that he ended up in a relationship with his roommate's ex girlfriend (they had all grown up together). I ended up sleeping with Jane's ex, to make Roy jealous (the A-typical child manoeuvre), and of course that served no purpose. She and Roy ended up together for many, many years to come, and had three boys. Jane and I became best friends after my first real boyfriend and I had split up (a few years later), but I was always a thorn in Roy's side. He wanted the proverbial house wife, meaning, he wanted her to stay home, and I wanted to go out and party. This caused a lot of contention between us, and I found myself eventually backing off for while.

Oh dear, now I am about to introduce you to the bar of choice, where I spent almost every day, whenever I wasn't at work. It was called the Scottsdale Inn, and the same place where I first met Roy. It was late 1979 to early 1980 when I started going there, having just turned nineteen years old. I met a couple of girls who befriended me, and ended up leaving home for the last time, and moving in with them. When one of them decided to move in with her boyfriend, I ended up living room and board with a great couple, Pat and Joan (I ran into Joan again at the race track this summer). They were really good to me. I had gotten a job at Glen River Industries, out towards Tsawwassen, go figure. We built mobile homes in the old airport hanger, and I was on the finish line. It was really strange to work there, and I was one of very few females that did. It was however, manned by all the "bad boy party animals" I had hung out with in Tsawwassen. The pool hall crowd, it was just like going back to school.

When I lived at Pat and Joan's (about 4 blocks away from the pub of choice!), I would have a nap as soon as I got home from work. Then Joan would wake me up for dinner, after which I would have a shower and head out. That was the daily routine. I am not quite sure, but I could not have been going there long before I met Leann. The first time we met she was absolutely polluted, and asked me if I could drive. Well, little did she know that I was just about as drunk as she was, and I told her "Sure, I drive?" "Would you mind giving me a ride home?" she asked, "so I can feed the kids, and then we can come back here?" "Absolutely, why not, bar's dead right now anyway," I told her. So, off we went. I got into the driver's seat of a car she had borrowed from another friend, and of course it was a standard. Well, never having driven a car in my life, I wouldn't have known a standard from an automatic anyway. All things considered, I probably only stalled it about a million times, but I got us home to her place. She made me admit that I indeed had never driven before, and she did drive back to the bar afterwards. We both had fun, and still talk about it to this day. Leann's husband was in a band and out of town a lot. She asked me to move in to help her with the kids (she had three), but all I really did was help us get plastered a lot. We ended up doing acid every day for about a year, before our supply ran dry. I remember sitting in the bar, unable to smile, unable to even force a smile. I realized then, that I could no longer have fun without the acid, and stopped doing it cold turkey. Just like that.

Dear Gosh, I thought I was done with this topic, but more and more great stories keep popping into my head. Leann and I did have a lot of fun together, I must say. Here's one...Leann's Uncle Kent was a major alcoholic, but he loved to gamble at the race track. Since he had to have his whiskey first thing in the morning when he got up however, he would take me along with him to the track. He gave me $100 bills (quite a bit of money at that time), and while he sat in the lounge, he would send me to go bet on the horses. He knew all the jockeys and we always came through the back way through the barns. He brushed me up on the game a bit, (about win, place and show), but I did not really know what I was doing. Served us well, for I had beginner's luck. To this day I am still good at playing with other people's money.

I never win with my own. Uncle Kent would give me half of whatever I won, and that was pretty lucrative. At about the same time this was going on, Leann and I got involved in the "Pyramid" scam. You would buy in at the bottom, which had eight squares... then four...then two, with one square at the top of the pyramid. The person at the top received the payout from all the eight people at the bottom. We both quit our job (which is a hilarious story, I will tell in a moment), to go to pyramid meetings. I received payouts a few times, and then they fizzled out, and I lost my money on the last couple pyramids. Anyways, between the pyramid money and the race track, I was able to pay cash for my first car. I woke up one Saturday morning, and called Uncle Kent to take me car shopping, and ended up with a gold Duster.

Oh yes, and the job we quit...great story this one, one of my favourites, actually. Leann and I decided to stop in at some random deli one afternoon, and along with some German sausages, I came out with a job for each of us. We started almost immediately, and the deli had a coffee shop attached, and between the two, there was a narrow hallway which led to a dining room, also part of the deli. We worked with a woman whom neither of us could stand, but she was the manager, since the owner was never even present. I cannot even recall his name. We called her "Gertie", however and she hated it.

Anyways, it was Halloween time, and Leann and I had a big party at the condo. It was a wild one, and we pulled an "all nighter." Prior to the party, we had been in some lounge one late afternoon, and Leann had noticed that someone had left their leather jacket in one of the booths. We decided to steal the jacket and took it home. It was later, when we had a chance to look it over, that we realized it was a Hells Angels' top members jacket, as it had the badge right on it. Needless to say, we ended up having a bonfire shortly thereafter, but not before we found some pills in one of the pockets. Stamped on the pills, it read "Upjohn 27," so we automatically assumed they were uppers. You know...something that would keep us AWAKE!

Well, we were both booked to work the day after our Halloween party, and not having slept at all, with a massive hang over, we were dragging our asses. We remembered that we had these pills, and had made sure to take them with us. When we could stand it no longer, we each decided to take one to wake us back up. The next thing I remember is someone ordering a milkshake. Since this company was too cheap to purchase one of those metal cups you are supposed to use, we had to make them in the cardboard cups they are sold in. Before I knew what happened, the stupid blade had drilled right through the bottom of the cup, and there was milkshake EVERYWHERE, and I mean EVERYWHERE! Gertie was not happy, and ended up burning her soup, whilst cleaning up my mess, since I was clearly unable. The next thing I remember was Leann shaking me awake, in the owner's office chair with my feet on his desk, sound asleep. Gertie had woken her up in the dining room and ordered her to wake me (because she could not) and we were asked to leave. Well...fired on the spot actually. Go figure! I hazily recall stealing a huge sandwich in front of her, and staggering out into the mall with Leann. I sat under the phone booth and munched on my sandwich while Leann tried to get us a ride. It turned out that the cab driver who showed up was a friend of ours named Smiley. Thank goodness he knew where Roy and Dale lived, and took us over there. Apparently, we were carried out of the cab, and distributed on the two couches in the living room.

That evening, everyone had gathered at the house as usual, and they woke us up to see if we wanted to go to the bar with them. After wondering for a moment or so if we could possibly handle it, one of us, I am not sure who, remembered that we had some acid. THAT ought to wake us up! The only problem was that when we much later got back to our condo, we were unable to sleep, of course, because that is after all what acid does. No worries, however, we still had a couple of those "Upjohn 27's!" When Al, Leann's husband came home from being out of town, the next morning...he was scared. He woke me up on the couch, completely freaked out because he had not been able to wake up Leann. We had to tell him the story.

# Chapter 2 - Along came Dennis

And now the toughest part for me to talk about...Dennis Vandill. Being the type of guy all the girls wanted, of course I fell in love with him. Jeez, guys, do you think there is a pattern forming here? I had previously met him in the bar. I always considered myself shy around men, although they don't agree, nor do my friends. I usually get what I want though, where men are concerned, and I snagged him. (Took me a few months on this one). I ended up going over to his house a lot in the next few months, and he in turn gave up all his other relationships. Shitty thing is he had come into quite a bit of money, after he got run over in the bar parking lot. Before long, Dennis became a full fledged junkie. Well...it wasn't long before he "turned me out," as we called it in those days. He introduced me to heroin first, I have never, and will never blame him for my addiction. I was irate though, when a short while later, he turned out his little brother, who ended up a chronic user, unable to stop. His brother ended up dying of Hepatitis C, years later.

After watching Dennis use the drug for a while, I begged to partake. The first time I had the needle put into my arm, I do not think I really got high. Sometimes that happens the first time or two. I can't remember who "fixed" me, for I could not do it myself, at first. Then you learn. It was intriguing and fascinating for me, to watch Dennis pull out the spoon, drop that white or brown powder into it, out of a little tiny capsule. Then he'd take the needle, suck up some water, squeeze a bit of it into the spoon, to dilute the powder. Next, he'd pull out the matches or a lighter, bring it to a short but rapid boil, drop in a small piece of filter (from a cigarette, preferably), and then suck the yellow liquid back into the needle. Oh, how I remember that sweet smell when you cook the dope. It almost makes me drool. Know I am literally salivating right now, just writing this.

Let me try explaining the high of heroin...when you release that golden liquid into your vein. First there is the ritual of giving that needle a little flick, as you hold it up to the light, to get out all the air bubbles (don't want those going to your heart), then you slowly puncture the vein, draw the needle back a tiny little bit (we junkies call this "flagging"), so it fills with a tinge of dark blood (that way you know you are inside the vein). The "feeling" hits you immediately, like about two to three seconds after you pump it into your system. It is a really warm, comfortable, fuzzy feeling. It engulfs your whole body, and in turn your mind. It hugs you like a lover cannot. Caresses you like none other. All the problems in the whole world dissipate immediately. It is really weird, even if you think of the bills you cannot pay or whatever it is that is plaguing you, it doesn't matter when you are high. I LOVED heroin, and I loved that my parents would hate me for doing all the bad things I did to myself. I could not get enough. I became a daily user as fast as you can spit on the sidewalk. They say, "It only takes one time to become a junkie...it will reel you in, no matter who you are." "It does not discriminate." I was hooked!!!

Life as a junkie...I have drilled it into my daughter's head her whole life, that there ARE consequences. You pay a big price when you abuse your body for as many years as I have. No one ever taught me that there were consequences. In my day, nobody really talked about these matters. The schools, media and parents were clueless. I was now beginning my twelve year long perilous path of being this person, who could not live without her drugs.

Not long after I started using, Dennis and I got an apartment together. Shortly after that, he quit working, and I paid all the bills for the next seven and a half years. Yup...dumb, dumb ass. Life was good, I thought at the time. The apartment building we moved into is still there and recently I ended up in the same complex. Talk about full circle! When we first moved in, I wanted to impress Dennis and make him an awesome dinner. I bought some potatoes and a chicken, looked at them when I got home...called my mom and asked her what I should do next. Since my mom never allowed anyone in the kitchen when she cooked, I didn't even know how to boil potatoes, and I am not exaggerating.

Remembering quite well one afternoon when a friend of ours whom we nicknamed "Pinhead," had come over, and proceeded to empty this huge bag of goodies onto our kitchen table. He had robbed a drugstore and we were set for many days. There was a very large variety of pills, clinical cocaine, Dilaudids (clinical Heroin), anything and everything. Strange though, when we were running out, I will never forget, Pinhead actually shot himself up with Gravol. I learned then, that there is something we call "Needle-Fever." Many junkies get more addicted to the needle, than to what is in it. I have seen people shoot ice water just to put the needle in their arms.

I think that all the drugs wore down our systems, because it was shortly thereafter, that Dennis and I went out for dinner one night, and both came back with food poisoning. We were severely sick for a good week...so sick we could not even do the dope, which made us sicker because our bodies needed it by now.

I don't remember how long we were in those apartments, or why we moved. I think it was just because this other place became available to us. We moved into a duplex beside a friend of ours in Surrey. We lived there for a few years, I think, but I am not sure how many. It was here that it became apparent to me, that Dennis was extremely abusive. Well, it was the hitting that I realized. I did not really understand the verbal and mental abuse, having grown up with it. I was raised to be very insecure.

Needless to say, over the years, Dennis had brainwashed me into believing I was a total loser. That I was unable to live without him, always running me down and calling me names. My biggest fear to this day is to be brainwashed in a relationship. I do understand completely why women stay in abusive relationships. They do not consider themselves worthy of anything better. It is absolutely true that mental abuse is much worse than physical abuse. I really believed that I could not survive without Dennis, which makes no sense to me now, since I was bringing in the pay checks?

I will never forget the Christmas he gave me a black eye. I was so scared of him, I didn't even fight back, just like with my dad. He told me that I was to tell our parents that I had banged my face on a cupboard door. "No way," I thought, "I cannot let him get away with it." I knew that I would be taking the chance of receiving another beating, by telling them all the truth, but I made sure to tell both sets of parents that it was Dennis that had given me the black eye. It didn't really change anything though.

Most of our years in that house are a blur to me. It was not long after we moved there (circa 1981), that everyone I knew (all our junkie friends, and there were many), ended up on the Methadone program. It saved everyone a lot of time and money. You see, aside from the heroin, we were heavily, (and I am talking about a daily habit), addicted to "Fiorinal," which is a really potent painkiller. The pills contain both codeine and barbiturate, and had the same sort of effect as the heroin. I took on average about ten per day, usually four or five, as soon as I got up in the morning. Everyone was doing them all the time, and it became a full time job to go "doctoring." The pills were so easy to get, all you had to do was tell the doctors that you get migraine headaches, which I had been plagued with since high school. In those days, there were no computer systems to keep track of how many doctors you had seen, or how many pills you had had prescribed. We all began exchanging medical cards, to hit up new doctors. The old cards only had a first character and your last name on them, so I became "Denise Vandill", and Dennis became "Peter Hoffmann." We had a good stash of pills at all times, but they were hard on the stomach. We also traded cards with all our friends. Oftentimes, a carload of us would go out doctoring together...and that could be a lot of fun.

I will never forget when Dennis's downtown doctor first put me on the methadone. It was just too easy. He started me on 35ml per day, and since I am a light weight (about 115lbs at the time), it got me so high the first time, that all I wanted to do was come down. I seriously thought I was going to overdose. Dennis talked me through it all night. Now the trick is that they want to saturate your system with this shit, so in order to stay on the program, I had to do this amount everyday. The first week was almost unbearable. One of the side effects, when you first start this drug is that you cannot sleep, so then the doctors also put their patients on Valium. I refused the Valium. I had seen my father go through withdrawals after his thirteen year Valium addiction. I remember him coming home from work many, many days, green, and puking in the toilet. The worst day I recall, was when he slammed in through the back door, marched into the living room, where we were gathered, picked up the stereo and smashed it against the wall, unprovoked and for no apparent reason. It was the anger that kicking this drug invoked, I think, that made him do that. I mean, we never wasted a single scrap of anything at home, my parents were so glued to their possessions.

After getting through the first week of Methadone, I felt better and better. It was not long before I asked the doctor for an increase and was eventually put on 65 ml per day for the next seven and a half years of my life. Had I not been an addict to begin with, and made sure that I was pumped full with drugs (because they make you take a urine test to prove that you are a junkie before they put you on the program), I would have overdosed that first day. A regular grown man can easily overdose on 20-30 ml of this stuff. Your body becomes saturated with it, and methadone is the only drug in the world that collects in your bone marrow. It is meant by the government to keep junkies off the street. Although at first it keeps you awake, it has the opposite effect when your system gets used to it. I have discovered that all hard drugs do this to you. The way they make you feel when you first start using, is the opposite of how they make you feel when you become addicted. Strange, but true, you can ask anyone who has been addicted to cocaine, or any other hard drug. Methadone, basically turns one into a couch potato.

We remained with a private doctor, in downtown Vancouver for a year, then the government realized that the doctors were abusing their rights, such as upping the doses too high, and of course adding in the Valium. We were then sent, to what at the time, was called the Foundation. There they had people in place that gave you your daily dose and made you drink it in front of them. The ministry wanted to make sure that the Methadone was not being sold on the street, which of course it always had been. For the first few weeks we had to go there everyday, and drink it in front of them. Then, only once a week, and they would hand you a weekly prescription. Once they allowed you a week to two week supply, you would have to leave a urine sample, to make sure that you were using it yourself, and that there was no street drugs in your system. With no stall doors in the bathroom, I used to get "stage fright."The best they could do then was run the water for you, because they had to watch you pee. You see, otherwise you could swap the piss. In other words, if you had abused other drugs, then you would just find a friend who hadn't done anything else and bring their pee in a container, and pour it into the cup. I have to mention here though, that heroin does not work together with the meth, the methadone overpowers it. Some people on "the program" sold most of their "juice" though, because they preferred to use the street drugs, and the methadone if used once a week would remain in their systems. Some of the people we saw all the time were pretty scary characters, many of them in and out of jail. Some had been in for murder, they told us. I am not sure how many years we had to go to the Foundation, but then the government began cutting back on funding, and the program had grown too large. We had to find a doctor out in the Valley, a good hour's drive away. All the doctors downtown were booked solid, and there were only so many doctors that were allowed to have their methadone licenses.

Back now to what I was saying earlier, there were many days and nights, that were so much fun, but, I can barely remember most of them. A couple more stories come to mind. Oh...oh, here is Leann popping into my head again...She and I had a falling out about one and a half years ago, over a real estate deal. She had actually told myself and everyone she knew and worked with that I had not bought her a present. She stated that other Realtors (get a load of this!) buy their clients major appliances and the such. Being the rebel that I am, I bought them NOTHING. I suppose that being a friend, and driving her to the hospital, during my work time wasn't enough. A couple of weeks after they had moved into their new residence, Leann totalled her car, and asked that I refer her to someone. She knew my financial situation at the time, and my struggles to keep food on the table for my daughter. She also knew that I would receive $100 referral fee from the salesman, since she blatantly asked. Leann also demanded that I give her half of it, and rather than start a war, I did indeed comply. So, I could not help myself, when I sent her and her husband a Christmas card that year with a $10.00 gift certificate to an East Indian Cuisine in their new neighbourhood. She does not like East Indians in the least, so I did not need to be a fly on the wall to picture her first sputter and spew, and then possibly laugh at the brazenness. We now talk again, as though nothing ever happened...an ongoing saga.

So, it must have not been too long after she and I met, that we had the crazy idea to have a bet over who could steal the most lighters by New Year's eve that year. It was a couple of months away. We came upon this idea because we were always ending up with other people's lighters in our purses at the end of the night. We diligently thieved all of our friends lighters, and for Christmas that year, I used an engraver I had had given to me, and on one lighter (the same colour I would have stolen from that person), I wrote their name, and on the other I printed their name. Then I wrapped them up in a toilet paper role, with a pretty bow on top. When I handed them all their Christmas presents, they said they felt bad because they had not gotten me anything...until they opened their gift!

Great thing was we got to steal them all back! One night, we were in the pub first, and then went next door to the cabaret, and lo and behold, there was a wet tee-shirt contest! Leann had this crazy plan, (because most guys crowd the stage for this "rare" event), in which we go to all the empty tables, and she would steal all the cigarettes, and I would take all the lighters, and then we would divvy them up. I thought that was a great idea. And so, we made our way through the entire lounge, and gathered so perhaps hundreds of lighters and packs of smokes. When New Year's had come and gone, Leann and I realized that we never did count out all the lighters in our boxes. We had a microwave size box each. We do not know for certain, although we think it had to have been quite close, who actually won.

There was one night, when a few good friend of ours, (four single guys, living together in a house) were going to have a party. Well, I guess I must have gone overboard at the bar, prior to arriving at the party. I was told later on, that I had been, not only kicked out of the bar, but barred from the Scottsdale. Ouch, that was my home! Leann and I later ascertained, from asking around, that it had something to do with me dancing on the pool table. Oops.

What I do recall quite clearly, (although only a small portion thereof) was actually, physically, oh so physically, coming through the back door of the house. The place was packed, and I proceeded to first draw the eyes of everyone in the kitchen and part of the living room upon me (I can be quite loud and boisterous), with my "Hi Everybody!" and no sooner had I said that, than I did a complete and total nose dive onto the floor right before me. Absolutely "gooned to the nines," I picked myself up as though nothing had happened, and staggered over to the table. There sat Fishin' Rod, and a few other really good friends of mine, but in the middle of the table sat a "60 pounder" of vodka and a "26er" of Kahlua! I was so...o...O happy, because I had been drinking Dark Russians (Kahlua and Vodka) and ordering a White Russians (with milk) to sip on, at the bar earlier. That was my drink venue at the time. Wait until you hear about the tequila days! Oh my...see, now I totally remember all the fun I had, fun, fun, fun, and more fun. That was the name of the game after all, until the drugs got a good hold of me later on, that is. And even then, there were a lot of fun times throughout.

So, let's go back to the part about getting saturated with the methadone, and the duplex with Dennis. Those were really crazy and blurry days. As I recall, sometimes not much happened, and only a few people would pop in and out to visit. I worked at Block Bros. Head Office (a real estate firm) at that time. I got the job through a friend of mine Janelle. Sometimes Dennis and I had parties, and quite a few people over, but mostly they just dropped by. They were all our user friends, meaning, they used drugs daily, just like we did. Dennis and I ended up together for seven and a half years, and I do not think he ever screwed around on me, but, our relationship was often very strained, and certainly not a loving, warm one. At the time it seemed normal, because my parents had not been warm and fuzzy either.

Looking back on it all now, I realize that our sex life was really fucked up. We did not have sex often (about once a week, I think), once we settled in, and he was not very good at it. I remember us only ever "doing it" in missionary position. The most creative he ever got was taking me from behind sometimes when we were drunk. I specifically remember one night, we were both really drunk, and he was taking me from behind, and he must have slipped...and that is how I experienced my first anal penetration. I still wonder if he knew, because we didn't ever talk about sex either. When I masturbated, I felt guilty, and would only take the chance when I knew he was out. I did not know how to take control, I was way too shy and inexperienced, so it was up to him.

Dennis was also five years older than I, and had slept with many, many women. This line up included, (I of course found out many years later) my own sister in law. When she found out who my ex was, she embarrassed me in front of the whole family, by relaying to me how small endowed he had been. She was right, you could barely feel the idiot inside you...but back then I wouldn't have brought it up in public that is for sure. Now, I don't care what anyone else thinks anymore. I think, at the time, we were together, the thing that I thought was the strangest, was that he absolutely refused to have a shower with me, claiming that he thought it was gross and disgusting.

Our neighbours in that duplex sure were entertainment at its finest though. It had turned out, that our neighbour was Dale's (my ex - Roy's roommate) older brother and his girlfriend Candy. Jay and Candy had been together about five years, and had a very torrid relationship. There was a lot of yelling and screaming next door, especially from him, and he used to beat the shit out of her on a regular, drunken basis. She was not allowed to go out or do anything without his permission, and this one day stands out so vividly in my mind.

Candy and I were sitting in her kitchen on a warm sunny day, and in came Jay, pissed to the gills. Somehow, he thought that she had gone out and was "slutting around," and he had this in his head, as he yelled and screamed in her face, and called her every name in the book. At the same time he had her by the back of her bleach blonde hair, and her huge boobs bounced up and down, right along with her head, as he rammed it into the kitchen floor, pulled her back up again, and rammed her head into the kitchen cabinets, over and over again. I kept screaming for him to stop, and when he finally heard me, his focus turned on me. He let her go, as she fell lifeless to the ground. He then began swatting blindly at me. I knew I was had, and turning tail, I bolted out the back door, down the three steps, through the gate and around the front, flying into my house.

Dennis looked up and saw the fear on my face, and quickly picked up a crowbar he had just been working with outside, when I told him what was happening. I begged him not to go over there, as Jay was completely out of his mind. I tried to convince him to call the cops instead. Now, you can only imagine how much we wanted the cops at our place with all the drug abuse and criminals always at our house. I really thought Jay was going to kill Candy that day. Dennis let me call the police. When they arrived, they came upon Jay standing in the driveway, hitting the ground with a baseball bat over and over again, coaxing them to just try and come closer. They knocked on the front door and told Candy that she had to press charges, for them to take Jay away. Candy of course fearing being killed later wouldn't dare do that. The cops stayed long enough, for him to calm down and leave the premises. That's when I learned it does not pay to get involved, after all.

Due to the fact that the years with Dennis are so distant, and the things I remember may not be in order, I will recall the times that stand out the most vividly in my mind. I recall that I worked and that when I was at work, Dennis would actually steal my "juice". The methadone was mixed with Tang orange juice, so that junkies would not fix it. We discovered however, that if you cook it in aluminum pots, you could get enough of the Tang out, to put it in your veins. These pots got so used, that they released a thick, grey murky goop that we then sucked up into the needle. That was the aluminum. I am afraid of Alzheimers now because of it. We didn't care then though and put it in our bloodstreams anyway. Sometimes, it had so much orange juice in it, that it would be really thick in the needle, and actually burned as you tried to pump it into your veins.

When I first met Dennis, his friends, (and he had many at that time) had him on a pedestal. He would have done anything for his friends, before he became a regular drug user. Now, they were losing all respect they had ever had for him. I remember the fights he had with friends, especially Fat Cat (our pet name [pardon the pun] for a dear friend), (who was in a wheelchair), because he would steal their dope, and they knew it. I actually saw him a couple of times myself, draw some of their juice right out of the pot with his syringe, while their juice was cooking on the stove. Before long, they stopped coming over, and of course, Dennis blamed me for it. He convinced me, (since he said it everyday) that I was such a bitch, (they had told him) that they did not want to come over anymore. He told me this so often that I actually believed it. The truth was, that we did fight in front of our friends a lot, and that made them uncomfortable of course. In fact, we fought all the time after a while, just like my parents had, when I lived at home.

I remember also, this one day, Dennis and I, had had a big blow out, and his best friend, (not a junkie) came and picked him up. As they were pulling out of the driveway, I had gone into the bedroom, and gathered a huge armful of Dennis's clothes. I ripped open the front door, and dramatically threw them as far as I could, all over the yard. Shitty thing was, that neither one of them saw me. Damn, now what was I going to do? Leave them there I guess, so he could be pissed off when he got back! Well, next thing I knew, it friggin' started to rain. Now I did not know what to do (obviously stoned beyond belief), because I knew who did the laundry, and it certainly was not him. In fact, when I lived with Dennis Vandill, he did not do anything. I did it all, and I worked full time. So, guess what? I went back out there, embarrassed now because I imagined our neighbours all to be laughing at me, and gathered the fucking clothes back up. Stupid, but that story always comes back to me when I think of the past.

Another night that really stands out in my mind in that house, was this one time that a couple of people (and I have no idea now who it was) came over, and they brought a shit load of cocaine with them. Since we were always into the "downers," but were out at the time, we decided to try to fix the coke. OH MY GOSH... what an extreme mind-blowing rush! Never had I experienced anything this dramatic before, anything that hit you so hard, and so suddenly. You see when you snort cocaine, it is quite a mellow stone, you do not even feel it the first time really. When you smoke cocaine, it amplifies the effects by about 1,000 times, but when you fix cocaine...OH MY GOSH! I recall sitting at the kitchen table, putting it in my arm, feeling stupefied and scared all at once, and quickly rushing to the couch, where I discovered the stereo blaring beside me, and my whole head, and ears were ringing. It was so unbelievably loud and amplified, that it actually scared the shit out of me. After that night, I only fixed the stuff one other time, in some flea infested trailer court with some unknown junkie I had met, and cannot remember what he even looked like. I knew people that did "speed-balls", which were heroin and coke together in the needle. I had heard that so many people overdosed this way, just like Belushi, so I refused to do it. Other than that, the only drugs I think I did not ever try is mescaline, and morphine, and PCP.

So now let us go into the part, when Dennis and I were evicted out of that house, which I really liked. What had happened was, that while I was at work, and having left Dennis to pay the rent and the bills, his habit had grown. He was now spending all the money I gave him for bills, stealing my prescription (because you had to keep it refrigerated, or the orange juice would go skunky), and before I knew it, our landlord was knocking on the door. That was how I found out that we were over two months in arrears, and that unless we came up with the money, he wanted us out. Since I did not have enough left for three months rent, we had to put all of our belongings (which other than one bedroom suite and the stereo, were all mine) into storage, and ended up living with some friends of ours, Abe and Jeanelle.

I worked with Jeanelle at Block Bros. head office as a conveyance secretary. She had been there first and was next in line, to the supervisor of my department. She had gotten me the job. I loved my job so much that I worked my way up the ranks in my department within two months, from mail and banking to just under Jeanelle. In fact the two girls that were already there when I arrived, were now doing my excess work, such as photocopying, etc. I was their boss, and of course they did not like that, and it was very awkward, since

I was still shy back then. Computers had just been purchased by large corporations, and the computer system we were on, was built by this old guy that worked there. He really liked me and took me to see the Mother Computer one day. He told me then that he had been in a German prison camp for years. He was Polish or Jewish or something like that, I am not sure. He led me into this room where right in the middle was this huge black box, about the size of a small bedroom. On one side of this box there were literally millions of threads, and he showed me that whenever anyone came on line, the computer would know this and "thread itself. It looked like one of those pictures they make in public schools, where you bang nails into a piece of wood and thread them like a Spiro graph. The system was so elaborate for its day and age, that a large company called "McMillan/Bloedel," who were in the same high rise downtown, where we were located, scrapped the brand new computer system they had just purchased, and came onto our system.

Anyways, I was taught on the computer, and in turn, it became a large part of my job now, to train all of the Block Bros. personnel right across Canada. I had to do this via telephone, so it was quite challenging. I was the one they called whenever they had any questions about the system. As it turned out, every year our supervisors had a meeting with management to negotiate the raises for their department. Kerry, my supervisor was completely gutless, and my department received the lowest pay increases in the entire company that year. Ben, one of the company's top managers, had luckily been watching my rapid progress, and called a secondary meeting with Kerry. He insisted that I deserved a larger raise based on my performance, and I ended up receiving the largest raise in the company that year. Alas, this did not bear well on Kerry, who was already afraid for her own job.

I can honestly tell you, and I have certainly told all of my friends and family over the years, that my job at Block Bros. was the best job I have ever had in my whole life. It is so true, I loved it there so much, not only because I was passionate about the job itself which was challenging, but because my hard work was recognized. Now other departments wanted me also. Unfortunately, Jeanelle and Kerry were jealous, and it was never to transpire.

This brings me to the part where, I lied to the company about why I was late for work every single Monday morning. Now, the methadone program being a government program, would have led to "wrongful dismissal," if it ever came out, and were to cost me my job. Due to my personal embarrassment about it all and Jeanelle's telling me not to tell anyone about it, however, I had to lie. The truth was that my job was downtown Vancouver, and the doctor I had to see to get my prescription (which we users called our "per"), was in Chilliwack. Since this caused me to be late once a week, Jeanelle and I came up with the story that I had a rare allergy, and that the only doctor who treated it was in Chilliwack. He even gave me a note to that effect.

So, as I arrived late again one Monday morning, I was stopped down in the lobby by one of the security guys at the front desk, and advised that there was an important phone call for me. "Strange," I thought, as I took the phone. It was Jeanelle on the end of the line, and what she told me next, shattered my life at the time. She proceeded to tell me that "they" had found out about my lie, and that "they" knew what I was really up to, and that "they" were hereby firing me immediately. Jeanelle told me that I should not bother coming upstairs to face anyone, and that she would take care of everything for me, and empty out my desk as well. I was so grateful that I would not have to look anyone in the eyes, and without ever turning back, I fled the building.

It occurred to me quite some time later, I have no idea when, or who may have said what to me about the incident, but I realized that it may have been Jeanelle and Kerry's way of getting rid of me. I had been feeling that I was about to receive a big promotion. I still often, think about how much I loved that job, and I have never found any other job to replace it. I have been searching my whole life since, and that was in 1986.

Not long before I had lost my job, Jeanelle had asked to meet me for lunch one day at work. I felt she wanted to talk to me about something important. This would have been in January of that year, because at Christmas time that year, Dennis had actually approached my father, sat him down, and asked for "his daughter's hand in marriage." So, when I met her for lunch, sure enough, Jeanelle wanted to talk to me about Dennis and me. She told me that she knew how unhappy and miserable I was, and talked to me about the constant fighting and bickering. I told her that because it had been more than seven years, the main reason I had stayed was that it had been such a long time, that I could not give up now, that I would be a failure.

Jeanelle somehow convinced me that day, that I could leave him, and that I was strong enough. She had slowly over time brought me to believe also that it was not my fault, that I was a good person, and that he had me completely brainwashed. It was as though something cleared for me that afternoon, and before I knew it, I went home and waited. I did not have to wait long, before I heard Dennis come through the front door, and I listened as he came up the stairs, my heart beating wildly. I noticed that he had a grocery bag in both hands (amazing he came up with five bucks!), and as he put them down on the kitchen counter, I told him that I did not want to be with him anymore, and that it was completely over.

Just like that, I had said it, I could not believe my own ears. Well...he must have believed that I was completely sincere, and without further ado, he picked up his grocery bags, (oh how fuckin' A-typical) and continued back down the steps, out the front door, and that was it! Viola...just like that! Well...he only came back to steal all of my stuff out of our storage. He cleaned it out bare, except for my personal belongings. Then the idiot had the audacity to phone me, and demand hysterically, that I give him back his bedroom suite his dad had given us. It was the better of the two suites we had. I still giggle over that! What an unbelievable moron...

Dennis was a pathological liar. Lying so much he himself couldn't decipher truth from fiction anymore. No one could tell. I ran into him about five years ago, and he hasn't changed an iota. As we said "Hello," I thought to myself, "you actually slept with this creep?" The typical regret procedure, and before I realized it he was already "storying" me. That's what he use to call it. He proceeded to tell me my dad made him leave me, because he had turned me into a drug addict. He told me that my dad filed charges with the police for his arrest. First of all, my father would never have the guts, and secondly he wouldn't have wasted his time and energy going through the procedure. Strange, how the brain works or doesn't work. Somehow, I knew poor Dennis absolutely believed that to be true.

Enough Now what? Mmm.m.m, I have to sit back and think for a moment...oh, yes...I cannot forget to tell you all about Rudy and Deanne. The two of them were a huge, huge part of mine and Dennis's life. What an interesting pair, I must say! For years we hung out with them almost daily. Rude and Dee were my parent's age... so that made them about 20 years older than myself. I am 48 now, mom's 70, dads 69, and my little brother Michael is 41. That makes my KK (whom you have not met yet...18.)

Rudy never worked a single day of his life. At the time all of their assets had been put in his mom's name. They had learned the hard way, after cops had kicked their door down more than once, and cut up every piece of leather furniture in the house, and demolished the rest. At one point, unable to prove how they had accumulated their wealth, the government actually seized their home, cars, boats, and every other asset they owned. Deanne was in and out of jail for most of their lives together. They had met, if I remember correctly, in their early 20's. Of course, this having been said, they had always been drug dealers. I keep forgetting not all of you automatically know this. Deanne, a big boned woman with the strength of a man, had spent a great deal of time in Vancouver's oldest and most dilapidated maximum security prisons called Oakalla. It has since been torn down, but the memories and the nightmares remain. “Word on the street” was everyone on the inside feared her. She would squash you like a bug if she did not like you. She ran the joint, so to speak. I went to visit her at Oakalla once, and it still seems surreal to this day. Through the glass with the phone, just like on TV. Creepy old place it was. I vividly recall Dee’s recount of the times she spent in solitary confinement. Once upon a time there had been a farm and cows there. Apparently, they put you in the old rat infested cow barns. In the winter, it was cold and damp, and she said they would slide the food trays under the door through a slot. I do not recollect any more of the specifics, I believe she had visited those barns quite often, and had found some intense inner resolve through her trauma.

Rudy and Deanne were extremely committed to each other, loving each other intensely, and they did everything together. They bickered once in a while, and sometimes he would be black and blue when we saw them. She finally admitted that she beat the shit out of him sometimes. He was just a scrawny, really skinny, medium height guy. You could snap him like a twig easily enough. Dee had a rough background, having been physically, mentally and sexually abused as a child. I’m not really sure, or remember what Rudy’s childhood story had been. She had worked on a poppy farm in Mexico at one point. She said that the fastest way to get high, other than putting the drug right into your bloodstream, was what they had done on the farms. They used opium suppositories. Interesting...she had also been in porn movies down in the States, I have no idea how many.

At one time she worked as a high class call girl to an elite clientele of five or six gentlemen. One was a doctor, one a lawyer, you get the picture. They all paid her $2,000+ a night, whether they just wanted her to join them for dinner, or whether she spent the night, the price remained the same, the way I understood it.

Deanne, who trusted no one, offered me this clientele on several occasions. She couldn’t really understand why I was unable to do it, but she respected my decision. I wanted to do it so bad, it sure would have fed all our habits, and the money at that time was unbelievable However, those damn morals my parents had raised me with, simply wouldn’t allow something like that. I thank my parents for those very powerful morals. Had it not been for those morals, or had I crossed the line even once, I would be dead today. I have no doubt about that. My belief system was so strong, I knew right from wrong, and the lines were heavily drawn, although in retrospect, they were not always right.

We used to go to their house a lot, and were definitely always there to fix, after we all picked up our pers. Dee would get us a "treat" every Monday, one we all looked forward to, all week long. Her doctor, who had a practise about ten minutes away, used to prescribe Dilaudids to Dee once a week, as long as she brought in some of her nylons, which he would then wear. I think they had sex, but she never really admitted nor denied that part. I think it would hurt Rudy. Dilaudids are a synthetic heroin given to patients who are in a deal of pain, such as cancer patients. They were done the same way as you did heroin. Crush them up in a spoon, add some water, cook the liquid until it turns clear, and then suck it up through a filter with the needle. Then you can go straight to Heaven.

Another thought that comes back to mind, I had never stolen anything from any shops, the entire time I was in school, and all my friends were shoplifting and daring me to do it too. When I started using the heavy drugs though, stealing stuff once in a while was so much fun. I remember one time when Leann and I walked into a store wearing shitty old thongs, (you call them flip flops now) and left the store with these cool burgundy coloured boots. That matched the burgundy hats we had just bought elsewhere.

These memories are returning because I remember Rudy wanting to take Dennis and the truck with him, whenever he was feeling energy, they would hit a strip mall. Rudy would go in, come out with a shopping cart filled to the rim with electronic equipment, load it into the get-away truck, (driven by Dennis) and off they would go. It was actually quite funny to watch. Did I mention that along with the money, Dennis stole from me that I left to pay the rent, he managed to steal and pawn off all my jewellery?

I admit I acquired most of it "hot." Our friend Jimmy would hire these young guys, and send them out to break into houses. This enabled us to get the jewellery really cheap. Dennis frequently went behind my back and pawned my jewels, and then he would get them back out of the pawn shop, over and over again, until finally he lost them. The one that hurt me the most was a necklace that my now dead Oma, from Germany, had had custom made for me. It contained a German Mark from 1865. It held a lot of sentimental value, and mom had often told me that she wanted to put it safely away for me, and I of course had refused.

# Chapter 3 - Alone for a Year

My life, from the time I kicked Dennis out, and before I met Grayson is another blur. I recall moving out of Abe and Jeanelle's shortly after Dennis moved out. Then I lived with a friend of a friend's, and her then 3 year old son, who ironically was Dale's kid, whom he never saw, or at that time even acknowledged. Dale was Jane's boyfriend, and Roy's best friend and roommate, whom I spoke of earlier. That worked out alright for a while, and then I remember my buddies, and I think my brother Matt coming over to help me move, but I will be damned if I can recall where the hell I moved to from there? I think I just had a basement suite after that.

Then I met Laura's niece Joyce. She was a piece of work that girl, I tell you. She was looking for a place and so she and I got an apartment together, a really nice corner unit on the bottom floor with a nice patio and treed yard. Joyce was the first person in my life that completely had me fooled, for I once was very good at reading people. I just wish I had always listened to my intuitions. I would have saved me a lot of time and money over the years. Ya, Joyce came across to everyone who met her as a totally sincere, but mostly completely naive and innocent, sweet young girl.

Turns out she was no such thing. The next thing I heard, although it took a couple months to come to light, was that she was sleeping with a major coke dealer. She would not come home for days at a time. Then I heard she had ripped him off for a couple of kilos of blow, but not until she had skipped town with the last two months rent unpaid, and a long distance phone bill threw me off my game I must say. I had to come up with all that money and fast. Real fast.

About the same time I had met and started hanging out with this big biker looking guy named Fred. I think I had met him through Joyce too, if I am not mistaken. He and I smoked a lot of crack together. Until then I had only smoked it a few times, and had only done rails (snorted it) on occasion before that. The biggest line I ever snorted actually almost killed me. I had gone over to a friend of mine's house for Christmas drinks one year. I remember Dale and a few other people being there, maybe six or eight of us. Teddy, a mutual friend had come over with his usual Christmas treat...a huge bag of blow.

I remember we were all in the master bedroom sitting around this big full length mirror they had laid upon the bed. They then proceeded to cut a line about 1/8 inch wide, and it covered the full length of the mirror. The next thing I knew, someone dared me to do the whole line, and everyone else chimed in, saying that there was no way I could do it all in one breath. Well...SOMEBODY had to prove them wrong...didn't they? Not proud to say, I did the whole thing, and the next thing I knew, my heart began beating out of my chest. Everything felt as though it were constricted. My breathing became almost laboured, and then the hugest wave of nausea I had ever felt enveloped me completely. I found myself tearing down the hall, someone close at my heels, and had barely gotten there before I found my head in the toilet. Wow, what a rush that was.

That reminds me too, of the times when you do a lot of heroin, you always puke. I could only ever go to see my parents when I was really high. I went out to Tsawwassen about three to four times a year to see them...and I would always get wrecked first. One time, Dennis must have had to pull over about eight or nine times on the twenty five minute trip out there, so that I could puke, I had done so much. My brother was seldom home whenever I did go there, and therefore I rarely saw him. I know my mom and dad wondered, and they certainly complained that I would talk incessantly the entire visit. That was because the pain killers, methadone and heroin made me talk a lot. Most people do the same thing on cocaine, but coke has the opposite effect on me. I have always joked about the fact that my friends used to like to give it to me just to shut me up. My parents though, were completely uneducated about drugs and alcohol, and because a beer bottle had fallen out of the back of our car once, they thought it was alcohol we had a problem with.

Alright, back to Fred, then. I hung out at his place quite a bit, there were always people over, and we were always trying to come up with enough money to "score." Fred and I also went over to Salt Spring Island quite a few times, because that was where he had grown up. I knew he liked me, but he was not my type at all. There was a younger guy who hung out at Fred's. For the life of me I do not remember his name. I still feel bad about it to this day, and this is one of my biggest regrets in life. He came over to my place one afternoon, and discovered I was a junkie. He was really curious about it and begged to try some. I held out a while, but finally broke down. Yes, I even put the needle in his arm for him and showed him how to do it. As I recall, he absolutely loved it. I still wonder to this day, if he is a junkie now. I'm sure after trying it, he chose it over the crack. The high lasts so much longer and it is cheaper. When you do cocaine, you are only high for about 10-20 minutes, and therefore everyone I have ever used with wants more. That is what they should have called it...MORE.

This brings me to my first (and only) arrest. While I was still with Dennis, we were always being tailed by "narcs" (narcotics officers). I cannot tell you how many times they pulled us over to search us, but we had horseshoes us our asses, we were lucky to never have it on us, and the methadone was of course, legal. The only time they took Dennis in and tried to charge him, was when they found a needle in his sock. He ended up in court over that one, because they found traces of heroin in the needle.

See, whenever they ran Dennis's name in the computer, he came up as a "suspected" drug dealer. As yet they had not caught him, and boy, did they try! That day, however, when they pulled us over, we had had a fight a short time earlier, and I "lipped off" the narcs, knowing full well that they would give him an extra beating. As he told me later, they did just that, saying "And this one is for your lippy old lady."

Another drama filled afternoon, occurred when we were over at a well known dealer's house, for a friendly visit, since he was a good friend of Dennis's. We were not there for much more than an hour, when the cops suddenly pulled into the driveway, giving Dennis no time to run, and so he had to swallow everything he had just scored. Again, they did not catch him, and since we had purchased the last of it, they could not arrest Skinner either. For those of you who do not know, when a dealer gets caught, and "they have to swallow it", that means that the heroin is wrapped up in balloons, which hopefully will not break in your tummy. If they break you would of course, overdose, and the way the balloons are later retrieved (in case you have not thought it through yet) is by shitting them back out. Gross or what?

A final cheque had come to my apartment, (Joyce's last work cheque), and she had just ripped me off. I thought I knew enough about her to go to Money Mart and cash it, and it took Fred a long time to convince me to do it. He drove me to Money Mart, I went in, and he said that he would wait out in the car for me. As I entered and found my way to the wicket, I tried to play it cool. I answered most of the questions without a hitch, and then something came up about who her dad was, and I suddenly came up blank. I fumbled my way through, making something up, and had myself convinced that I had done okay. They asked me to have a seat in the waiting room along with a couple other guys, while they confirmed the information. I was a bit nervous to say the least. You know, I have always taught my daughter to always follow her gut feeling, and to go with your instincts, even if it seems ridiculous sometimes. Wish I had followed my intuition and gotten the hell out of there that day!

The next thing I knew, I heard the sirens, and of course, they pulled right into Money Mart. There was one station wagon, which I and the other guys in the waiting room noticed had two dogs inside, and then there was a marked car with another bloody dog inside. "Shit," I thought, (they must be here for one of these guys,) facing complete denial head on. I looked at them and they at me, and I did not know what to do. We all wondered out loud what was going on, but we did not have to wonder long. The officers came directly for me, and asked me to come outside with them. I have never been more embarrassed in my life. (Well, not since the time I woke myself up on a bus, due to the fact that I was snoring so loud, whilst drooling on a perfect stranger's shoulder. When I awoke, everyone on the full bus was staring at me, and the guy whom I drooled on, had been too shy to pull away, was now turned beet red.)

Before I knew what happened, I was in the back seat of a cop car. The officer was super nice asking if I had ever been arrested before. I told him "no." He went on to explain to me that what I had done was called "fraud," and did I understand what that meant? I had no idea, and told him about Joyce and the cheque, through my tears. He told me that fraud is one of the worst charges to be up against, and that they were taking me to the station and finger-printing me, etc. I will never forget the way I felt when he pulled up to the cop shop, and was walking around the car to let me out. All I could think of was running, I was so scared. It didn't even matter to me that those dogs were there, I really considered it. I was so afraid. I didn't have any idea what would happen to me next. I got finger-printed, and after the paperwork was complete, they released me.

The matter was due to be handled in court, and in the mean-time I had to see a court appointed counsellor twice a week, and later once a week. The counsellor believed I wasn't really a criminal, and had just done something stupid. When the matter was up to go to trial, the counsellor told me that the police officer believed in me. He had apparently met with the judge on my behalf, and had begged me off. Since the courts were so backed up at that time, the charges were dropped. I always wished I had thanked that officer. Makes me wonder how many times someone just like myself actually ends up in the system, then really DOES became a criminal, thinking they now have nothing to lose. I was so lucky!

# Chapter 4 - Life with Grayson

After that, my friendship with Fred soon fizzled out. I put an ad in the newspaper for a new roommate. This strange fellow, Guy moved in. He worked during the day, came home, went to his room, and once a week he had his buddies over to place dungeons and dragons. Round about this time, I had met another group of friends, who all hung out together, and one of them was this guy named Kurt. Kurt really liked me, but he was a total alcoholic, and was really crass and low class, (although I hate to judge.) Anyway, this one night Kurt took me over to a friend's house. I distinctly remember walking into a huge rec room, and up at the bar, perched on a stool...there he was.

I knew instantly that it was what they call "love at first sight!" The rest of the evening is a haze I recall playing pool. Now, the thing is, I didn't want to hurt Kurt's feelings, and did not know how I was going to do it yet, but I just had to see this guy again! That is all I knew. I learned quite quickly that he was single, and before we left, sitting up beside him at the bar, I asked him if he would be up for a date with a friend of mine. Either that or he had asked me if I had any friends he could meet? Ya, I think that was it. I told him about Mandy, and that she was out of town at the moment. I asked him for his phone number and I gave him mine. I suggested he call me in a couple of days, and find out if she was back in town, and I would hook them up. Kurt noticed nothing, and I believe that was the last time I went anywhere with him.

Lo and behold, Grayson called a week later. I vividly remember sitting on the edge of my bed when he called, and my heart was pounding ten million miles an hour. He asked about my girlfriend, and I told him that she was still out of town. "But," I said, "I'm not busy, why don't we go out and do something together?" "I thought you were with Kurt?" asked Gray. I assured him that I was not with Kurt. I wish I could remember where he took me on our first date, but all I know is that we were inseparable after that. We spent every minute we could together. I was still working at Revenue Canada then. At that time in my life, if I really liked a guy and thought we would create a lasting relationship, I did not want him to think I was promiscuous. It was my personal rule to wait two weeks before I would have sex with them. That did not include one night stands or casual relationships. It is only very, very recently that I have admitted to myself that I have been a bit of a slut all my life. In my convoluted mind, I had myself convinced that I did not sleep with that many men. In actually though, I cannot put a count on it, because I do not remember a lot of my encounters. I do know that when I am with someone I love, I become a sex-a-holic of sorts. I love sex so much, and just like a man, I think about it all the time. Well, only when life is good though. I have had a couple of bouts where I was completely celibate for a year at a time.

So, knowing that I was completely in love with Gray, I made us wait the two weeks, right to the very last minute. It was really, really difficult. Sex with him was fantastic. Gray is the man who taught me how to overcome my inhibitions, which is what I had always used drugs and alcohol (especially alcohol) for. I know that a lot of people drink more when the relationship is new. After we got to know each other intimately, we ended up both taking a week off and stayed in bed for the whole entire week! We only got up to go to the bathroom or make something to eat. Gray is also the man who taught me how to cook. That was a damn fine week if I do not say so myself!

What I have also neglected to tell you about is that after Dennis and I split up, I became a party animal once again. Just like the old Scottsdale days. It always bothered me if I had to go to work or something, and my friends had a party without me. It drove me nuts actually. Oh, and another one is how I got the job at Revenue Canada. I had owed them some money and they had been looking for me for a year or two, but since I had moved around so much, Revenue Canada had lost track of me. I thought, "Wouldn't it be funny if I worked for them?" and with that I applied and got the position. They were looking for me and I was working right under their noses. What a hoot! I ended up working there on and off for the next thirteen years. It was only seasonal at that time though and eventually I would want something more, but that will come.

Oh, I have got to tell you this funny story. And what a small world it really is sometimes. I had been with Gray for about a month or so, when I got up one night to go for a pee. As I left the bedroom, I noticed a dim light in the kitchen. Curious, I went to check it out, and came upon a strange sight! There was a naked man standing profile in the light of the open refrigerator door, drinking pickle juice straight out of a jar. I froze mesmerized and wondered if this was perhaps a dream, and I was still sleeping? Putting down the jar, he noticed me standing there. As he turned on the kitchen light, he recognized me. "Petra!" he shouted. "J.T.," I shouted back, "what the fuck are you doing here?" What a surreal moment in time. Jay Ruddler (J.T.), was a good friend of mine whom I had met many years ago through Dennis and his friends. Turns out that J.T. used to be Gray's roommate, and he and his wife had had a fight or something and there he was, naked in the kitchen of my boyfriend's house drinking pickle juice! I still drink pickle juice, and have gotten many questioning looks from people. I found out later that when one has a stomach ache, drink pickle juice. It totally relieves gas and works really fast. That is pretty much what gripe water is, and that used to be what we gave babies when they had gas.

It is super important to me here to tell you something, before I delve any further into the Gray saga. After having known him for almost two weeks, and before I slept with him, I sat him down at the dining room table at his house. This was really hard for me, and I had agonized so much about having to tell him this, that I lost so much sleep over it. It is still to this day, so very hard for me to bring up sensitive issues, even so simple as asking for a raise. I really do not handle rejection well. Gray, of course knew that something was up and seemed genuinely concerned. I don't recall how I finally managed to blurt it out, but as we sat at that dining room table which would become so very familiar to me, I told Grayson Kelly that I was a junkie. I truly believed that he would dump me like a hot potato right then and there, because this was a man with a lot of class. Not that I did not have class, but what is classy when you are a filthy junkie? I waited, holding my breath...

I will never, as long as I live, forget his response, no matter what. He looked deep into my eyes, and all he said was "Do you want to quit?" Those became the most important words of my entire existence. Without any hesitation what-so-ever, I told him and I knew in my soul that, "Yes, I want nothing more than to quit doing this to myself." His next words were even more poignant... "Then I will help you," he said all matter of fact.

I could not believe my ears, I really honestly could not believe what I had just heard. "Don't be ridiculous, do you have any idea what you would be getting yourself into?" I questioned. "If you were smart, you would turn tail and run as far and as fast as you can, right now!" "If you are truly serious, and you really want to quit, I will be here every step of the way," he responded. I wanted to be happy, and I was, I was happy, but a part of me also thought that this was just too good to be true. I tried then, to explain to him just how fucked up I really was, but he did not seem to care. I knew then beyond a shadow of a doubt that this man truly, sincerely loved me, for who I was, and not what I had done. I could not believe that a guy of this calibre seemed not to judge me on any level. I can honestly say that Gray never judged anybody. Even I, although I try so hard not to, find myself judging others sometimes.

And, I will have you know, as time went by, and it was a long and difficult process, Grayson James Everett Kelly never wavered from his initial commitment, even when I did. Oh, how I recall the hell I put him through. I made it a rule in my life then, and I still do the same to this very day...I gave him "an out" all along the way. I must have done so every couple of months...I kept reminding him that there would be no hard feelings. If he wanted to back out at any time, I would totally understand. I certainly would not have blamed him, for I did not know if I could have done the same for another human being that he did for me. It was completely selfless. He became my Knight in Shining Armour, so to speak, but I also understood later on, that that was what Gray needed. He was addicted to "The Damsel in Distress." Funny how we are drawn to certain people in our lives. It turned out later that he was a super control freak, but with no bad intentions, just a control freak, like his Mother.

From Gray I learned a lot, and the funny thing is that it was one of the happiest times in my life, even with the hard work ahead. I felt completely loved and protected by him. Nothing at all like Dennis, where even though I was with him, we were never really present. All we ever focused on was how to be and to stay high. It becomes a full time job and obsession, because to be sick is so horrible. Neither one of us was ever truly "with one another" since the drugs were the most important thing.

My contract was about to run out at Revenue Canada, and I was about to lose the apartment, because my roommate had given his notice. He was moving in with a friend who had recently split up with his wife. And so, it was only about two months after we met, before I moved in with Gray. It was a massive house, and he had had two other roommates just before that. One of them, Mack, I think was still living there, but moved out shortly thereafter. Slowly, over time Gray taught me how to learn to love and believe in myself. No one had ever had that sort of an approach with me before, and I began to believe that I could actually do this. I had always told my friends that I needed to find someone or something more important to me than the drugs. I had also said that I had to find this before I turned thirty years old, otherwise I knew that for myself I would succumb and die doing the shit. Fat Pat Cat (as we lovingly called him) later died of Hepatitis C. I got the blessed opportunity to say goodbye to him in the hospital.

Imagine it really, when you are on "the (methadone) program," you cannot even leave the country. It is like a ball and chain around your ankles all the time. When you sell too much or do too much on the first day or two, you end up really, really sick, for the rest of the week. I mean physically sick. It kind of feels like you have a really bad flu, but worse. You get all clammy, you have night sweats, shivers, headaches that would blow your mind, intense nausea and vomiting, cramps, muscle aches, bone aches, stomach aches beyond belief, even your hair hurts. I will never forget the trips to go to the doctors or the foundation on a Monday morning, sicker than a dog, practically crawling to the car (you get so weak). Then if it was a sunny day, my eyes would hurt and tear so badly, because they get really sensitive to the light when you are "dope sick." How we used to race home to fix, talk about speeding. See, even when you drink "the juice," it takes up to about an hour to kick in sometimes, just like when you take a pill.

Since Gray wanted nothing more than to be with me whenever and wherever possible, he would sometimes tag along when I picked up my prescriptions. and then headed over to Rudy and Dee's to fix afterwards. I became so comfortable with him and he with me, that I did not mind him tagging along. Rudy and Dee, who had no other friends to speak of, must have truly trusted him also, and they trusted no one. One day in particular springs back to mind. It was one of those Mondays when I was really, really "dope sick." These trips and the waiting were complete agony. In pain, we raced back to Rudy and Deanne's so that I could fix.

Dee and Rudy were in the dining room at the table where they had cooked their stuff. I ended up in the bathroom because I already knew I was going to have problems fixing. See, by this stage, I did not have any veins left to inject myself in. I have always had very thin and small veins in my body to begin with. The orange juice that remains in the methadone after boiling and filtering it, causes your veins to collapse. The long term, continued use of any drug that is injected, also causes one's veins to collapse. The orange crystals however, accelerate the process.

I had just made it to the "can" with the cooked product and had gotten it into the needle, when Gray began knocking on the door. I tried really hard to ignore it, but he kept knocking. When I finally answered the door, I was in a sweaty frenzy, and totally exasperated. Gray begged me to let him come in. "I do not have time to deal with this," I thought, and ordered him to go away. He would not give up however. He told me that he would rather come in there with me and endure what he was about to see, than to be even more uncomfortable witnessing Rudy and Dee doing the same thing out there. So, desperate to just get the shit into my system, I hurriedly let him in. I sat up on the counter, and tried and tried to hit a vein with no success. I must have stabbed myself so many, many countless numbers of times. Finally, sweating and shaking, I broke down in a panic and tears. I did not know what to do, and the fact that Gray was actually watching all of this made me feel like the lowest parasite in the ditch of life. (How he must have seen me), I thought. He did not know what to do or say, either, but he managed to calm me down. He told me that it was all ok, and to take my time, and try again. He actually understood, which as I have learned throughout my life and all my addictions, is virtually impossible for persons who have not actually ever done the exact same thing, in the same way as I was struggling with. I hope that all of this makes any sense at all, because it does to me. That is why I am able to listen to and help so many people now. I have walked it and talked it and lived it. Whenever I expected Gray to judge me, (because I would for a moment see me through his eyes), he did not. I really looked up to him for being capable for such a feat.

As time went by, and after getting to know me better and better over time, we talked about me slowly weaning myself off the juice. That is to say that I would do a few milligrams less each week, cutting it down by 5 milligrams per week. You know, the methadone program was originally set up and described by the government, to get junkies off the streets and living a normal life. Their goal was supposed to be to wean everyone off of the methadone, once they had them levelled out at their prescribed dosages. Well, the weaning off part never, ever, happened that I was aware of. The only time a doctor did this with their patients, was when the patient asked to be weaned off. Only, everyone would always get too sick along the way and increase their doses again. The odds of getting off of the methadone bears a statistical success rate of .5%. Yup, not 5%...but point 5 per cent. That is why so many addicts do not ever even bother to try. I have known friends that have been through detox 9 or 10 times, and some even more than that, and still not get clean.

Well, the weaning myself off didn't work for me either. Whenever I did do less though, I sold the rest. At that time, you got $1 per milligram. I have no idea what it would be worth these days. That was potentially $420.00 per week, which was nothing to sneeze at. Funny, though, as honest as I thought I was being with Gray, I always fell off the "weaning wagon," and lied about it. Whenever he went to work or something, I would pull out the pot, and cook more. I even had a torch hidden in the bedroom, and would sneak an extra fix every chance I could. He caught me a few times.

A memory stands out so very, very, vividly. It was one of my most drug addicted humbling moments of intense insight, seeing exactly what I did not ever want to witness. My own fucked-up-ness

I call it. It was like looking in a mirror. I had never really been able to look at myself. It was not until about one year ago, as I sat on the toilet at my brother's house one night, after a few drinks. Right beside the toilet is a mirrored glass shower door. I looked over and suddenly had eye contact with myself. Unlike before, I maintained contact. While I was maintaining eye contact with myself, and finding it harder and harder with each second, I realized that this was the first time in my life, I had ever done this, EVER! Friggin' 48 years old and never been able to look myself in the eyes! Was it because I always knew I was also a liar, and disliking liars so much, not ever being able to admit it to myself? I have discovered that my entire family is a construct of lies built on more lies. My mom and dad, my brother and his wife, they all lie, all the time. They lie so much, they do not know that they lie. They lie so much that they do not know fantasy from reality. Just like Dennis. Well, it occurred to me recently that I also, have spent an entire life lying to people about who I really was. I lied to doctors, I lied to employers, I lied to family, and to my straight friends. And certainly, I lied to myself. All those vain years and hours putting makeup on in the mirror, could this be true? Wow, mind blowing...

Anyway, Gray had left one morning, for work, a normal morning, just like any other. As soon as he was out the door, I knew I was good to go. He was driving a big rig, and so I knew that if he found an excuse to turn around and come back for any reason (such as catching me fixing again), I would hear the truck. I wasted no time, as I was practically panting for this fix. After all, when you are weaning off the crap, and doing less and less, you never get "high" anymore. But then, when you do extra...viola, a rush, a warm glow. That wonderful feeling I've chased my whole life, that in reality isn't all that great anymore. It is all really what you imagine, in anticipation of the fix. Very seldom does it affect you the way it did when you first started, but that super rare, odd time, is what we remember, and keep striving for. The thing that keeps us coming back for more, and more, and more.

So, I had already stashed the pot and the outfit (another word for needle) and the filters and spoon and all that I needed, under the kitchen sink. I bent over to pull it all out, and had it all propped up on the stove. I was almost finished boiling it, when all of a sudden I heard someone coming up the back stairway to the small landing outside of the kitchen! No one ever used that staircase or doorway for shits sake. I panicked, there was no time. I grabbed the needle and the spoon and stuff, and tossed them under the sink, but I could not waste the precious dope, and it was still hot. So, I conveniently, and ever so nonchalantly, just stood in front of it, as the fuckin' door actually OPENED! Ah.h.h., he had thought ahead and had already unlocked the door. The prick (and of course he was the bad guy now, in my little head), had parked the semi down the friggin' road so I would not hear it, and had the audacity to SNEEK up the back stairwell, which nobody ever used. And for what? To catch me doing absolutely nothing at all, of course. Yup, that is correct folks. I stood in front of my pot, all pompous, my arms crossed and my back straight. I totally and utterly DENIED to his FACE that I was cooking any dope, or doing anything wrong at all, whatsoever! And it made all the sense in the world to me at that moment. Shit, I even had myself convinced there was no dope, no pot, no spoon, no nothing.

I honestly do not know why he stayed with me throughout all this. Our relationship endured so much, Grayson endured so much. He loved me so unconditionally, but I still do not understand how he did it. He must have felt so utterly helpless sometimes, especially when I turned it around, and I would be mad at him for ruining my life, just like a child. I mean how dare he fuck up my high? Well, that and a few more like it, were the last straws, to convince me that I could not do this on my own.

It was February 1989 the first time I went into Detox. Gray and I had been together since 1987. He always had a way of making these sorts of things seem like they were my idea. He had had two years to teach me how to believe in myself enough, to make the call to rehab. It is as though you know in advance that your best friend is about to die, and you have to pull the trigger to put him out of his misery. I do not remember the exact day that I picked up the phone to call them, or if it was me or Gray, who initially made the call.

All I could hope for was that they would have a bed for me right away. I knew for a fact from my junkie friends, that if there was a waiting period, which sometimes there was at that time (it is a lot worse of course now a days), then I would just get really, really high, and that would be that. An addict cannot afford to wait for a bed. If there is no help at the time an addict breaks down and makes the call, it is forgotten about and denied again forever sometimes. I was a bit luckier, they told us that there would be a bed available the next day, and we made an appointment. Of course, that day I did as much as I could without overdosing, I just wanted to get wasted for the last time. It seems to be an automatic junkie response, we need that last fix, no matter what.

I think though, at that particular time, that I languished more in the memory of what is was like when I had first started using. You know, that feeling that envelopes you every once in a blue moon if you are lucky, and for some people who are happier, I suppose the feeling hits them more often. But, you know that feeling that hits you when say, you are driving down the road, it is a beautiful, sunny day, the stereo is blasting your favourite song, a smile you cannot wipe off your face is plastered there, you look up at the sky, and you know that everything in that moment is right with the world. That warm, cuddly, vibrant feeling that encompasses, and caresses every nook and cranny of your entire body both inside and out. It holds you close for a long time if you let it. Well...that is what it is like the first while. Don't ask me when it slowly subsides without your even noticing, but that is what using opiate drugs is like. It is the best euphoric feeling in the world, because that feeling of being sublimely at peace with the whole world is amplified even more by the drug.

So now, I was having drug induced memories of how great my dope had been for all those years. And, why, exactly did I want to give it up? Oh, yes, I remember, in order to live longer. And, I really was in love with Gray and wanted to have a baby with him in the worst way. For, you see, I had been watching him for quite a while now. I knew beyond a shadow of a doubt, that Grayson Kelly was the epitome of the best dad I could imagine for my baby. My step son, Braydon, is 22 now, and I have known and loved him since he was one year old. We had him every second weekend, and Gray was honestly the best father I had ever been privy to. Gray is all about family. He had a lot of friends, but only held a few close, but never too close. The rest were only acquaintances who loved to party. You see, Gray had been the youth that had gotten kicked out of every school in Surrey (Canada's largest municipality at the time, and now a city). He was the class clown, and obviously disruptive. He was the life of the party, and together we were unstoppable.

So, now it is February of 1989, twelve years of daily drug abuse later. And Petra Hoffmann of all people, is off to rehab. Maple Cottage rehab. Unbelievable! I do not really recall arriving there, and I wish Gray was here to answer all of my questions, but I think it was really early in the morning. I suppose I had to have been up all night. It wasn't a bad place. I think they took us to the living room first and introduced us around. Then they took all my credentials probably, and showed me to my room, after I had said goodbye to Gray. All just guessing here, mostly. I think I had to stay for a minimum of ten days, and Gray was not allowed to see me for the first week, or something like that.

The next thing I recall is perhaps couple of days later. I wake up in my bed, and I am in pain, and feeling really sick. This is not fun, it is not fun at all. The next five days were spent in bed, writhing like an animal, in and out of delirium. Sweating, stinking, cold, in pain, vomiting, in pain, every muscle, ever bone, my head, my body, more vomiting, more excruciating pain. They gave me a medicine called clonidine, which lowered one's blood pressure to an almost non-existent level. This lessened the pain as much as possible, and prevented you from harming yourself. It slowed down everything, and especially time. Time had never, ever, ever, gone so slowly! You see, aside from all the other anguish, when you are drug sick from methadone, you do not sleep. Not one friggin' measly little, bittle, little wink. Not one!...for five days, no sleep. Can you imagine that? The only thing that I remember kept me going and even wanting to breathe just one more long, anguishing second, was what a really good friend (who had just been through detox) said to me. He had not slept himself for eight days. He told me, and I believed him (now I know it not to be true), that "no one has ever died from lack of sleep." It was the only thing that kept me going.

In case you think that part is bad...let me go on. After day five, they made me get up at 5 am to be at the breakfast table at 6 am sharp. Hell...pure utter hell! Sicker than a dog, wanting to puke, and roll into a ball, I had to drag my sorry ass (looking like shit warmed over), into that Gosh forsaken lunch room. There I was faced with a bunch of strangers, some very good looking, (I might add to my horror). It did not matter that I had eaten nothing I could recall in five days, or whether I could even stand the stench of the place. I had to be there. To make matters worse, I was supposed to drink fuckin' prune juice. Talk about beat a dog while she is down! That continued for a couple of days. Afterwards, rather than let me go and die in my room, they made me mingle and go to their stupid little meetings. They were actually quite interesting, when you weren't too caught up in the pain to listen for a moment. I do not understand why exactly, but whenever I am in pain, I feel intense anger.

It was the second or third day out of my room, that one of the staff members screwed up royally. They said that I was on some cockamammee list to go on some walk around Queen's park with a bunch of other yahoos, I was "doing time" with. I begged and pleaded for them not to make me go, saying that I was still way too sick, but to no avail. Well...the walk was the longest I can ever remember, it literally almost killed me. They made me keep going, until up the last hill, I completely collapsed. I almost ended up in the hospital, and found out soon after that I had not been on the list at all. It had been way too soon.

To this very day, I hate walking. If a store is half a block away, I get into my car. Anyway, I think I stayed in detox for about a week. I do not think I made it for the ten days minimum that they recommend you to stay. Grayson came and picked me up and took me home. I made it through the next couple of weeks, and it was really, really difficult. The thing of it was that I was still picking up my methadone prescriptions. I had it in my head that I could now sell all of my juice and therefore have an added income of $420.00 per week. That was a lot of money in the 1980's. Looking back now though, I don't even think I made it two more weeks "without." I talked Gray into letting me do like five milligrams a day "just to take the edge off" so that I was not sick anymore. That worked like a charm, but then of course, it went up to ten mils and day, and you can probably figure out the rest for yourself. Before I knew it, I was not selling it anymore.

So, then, let's talk about the second time I went to Maple Cottage rehab. Weird, there was a huge fire there that I caught on the news about 4 weeks ago now. The first time in there would have been in February, and the second time was in July, I believe it to be July 6, 1989. I think that I have trouble recalling my "clean date" because I know in my heart that I have never really been clean. Maybe I will never be, but if that is to be my choice, then that it my choice. I will tell you now that I must be ok with it. I know I have said this before, but so many people I try to explain that to just do not, cannot understand.

I was sitting on the couch in the "living room," when this woman was wheeled in. She had been dead on arrival at the hospital, after having a terrible wrestle with alcohol. She had been shipped straight through from the there to detox. There was also an older guy there, I think he arrived a day or two earlier. He was an alcoholic having been shipped straight from the hospital as well. I will tell you this, I have never in my life witnessed two individuals sicker than those two people were. They went through the DT's so bad, no television show had ever prepared me for this. They had seizures, blackouts, puking, screaming, shakes, and convulsions. It was a traumatic sight.

Excessive alcoholism, (for I learned there that there are many types of alcoholics) the ones that drink hard stuff from the moment they open their eyes in the morning, man, they go through hell, like no other addicts. And you know what they both told me? I spoke more to the woman, who confided her life story to me, but they both shared with me that they had no intention of quitting. They told me that as soon as they were out they would head to the nearest bottle. They had both been through this so many times before, and believed that they could not quit. The trouble in these situations became clear to me after the woman explained it all a little more. She especially, like so many others, have nothing more to look forward to in their lives. Many are old people that have to die and leave this world all alone, for they have no friends and family left to hold them up. It is like that, they have nothing and no one else, so it does not matter to them if they die tomorrow, as long as they die drunk.

When I left rehab about two weeks later it was with a different mindset than the first time around. The hard part had just begun, however. This long, long road became the steepest I have ever climbed. Next came the counselling and the meetings, but not before I was so sick, that for the next six months I could not even wash my own hair. Gray would have to come into the bathroom, where I would be perched in the tub, for I was too weak to stand in the shower. He would physically wash my hair, for I could not keep my hands raised up long enough to do it myself. You know, that feeling, that some women may have experienced from time to time, when they are doing a special hair-do that takes a long time? Your hands raised for so long that they become so tired, it feels as though they will fall off?? That feeling.

I honestly felt as though I had a violent flu for at least six months. I could feel the methadone actually drawing out of my bones. It was excruciating pain, to have to undergo this. Methadone is the only drug in our worldly existence that gets right into your bone marrow. It hurts like hell when it escapes your system. It is said that Hitler's doctor is the one who invented methadone, and that is how Hitler kept his army under control and faithful to him? He had the entire army strung out. And isn't it ironic, don't you think, that the government uses methadone to this very day to control junkies?

It is very difficult to describe to you just how sick I truly was for the next while, after detox. I just spent a lot of time on the couch watching television. It was difficult, to say the least. Thank Gosh I had Gray to take care of me. There is no way that I would have ever been able to accomplish this on my own. Grayson Kelly saved my life, the way I see it. And not just that, but the great guy that he was, he rewarded me with a trip to Mexico. I have never travelled anywhere, since my early days in Germany. I was so excited about that trip, and the flight alone thrilled me. Needless to say the night before the trip neither one of us slept. We were like two little school kids.

So, off to Mexico we went! Upon arrival we went first to the restaurant/pub that was downstairs from our hotel room. We had only one or two drinks since we were so tired...it had been about 36 hours since we'd slept. I used to have a gorgeous sunset picture of the two of us the waiter took that night. Our hotel was nice, it was a 5 star. Our suite had two bedrooms, kitchen, a living room, balcony, and a huge twelve man dining room, along with two bathrooms. I have no idea why we ended up in such a large suite, but who was complaining? Talk about being pampered!

Up to this very date, (and this is true) I have never in my life had a more fun-filled week. It was the best week of my life. What really made our vacation, (and I highly recommend this to anyone) is that we met a local girl almost as soon as we arrived. We first met her in the lobby of our hotel, where she worked there making sure that everyone was comfortable and had everything they need. She then invited us to join her and her crew aboard one of those cruises, where they take you to an island that you can only get to by boat. Alba and her blonde bombshell of a friend were hosting this vessel. On board we met the rest of our fellow vacationers, most of who were also at our hotel. Needless to say, this was a day and a night I will always remember.

We got to this gorgeous little tropical island and there was a grass hut with a full bar and kitchen, surrounded by lounge chairs and tables. The next thing we knew, there was a fashion show, and in it were both of our hostesses! It was the first time I had been introduced to a sarong, and they modelled 100 different ways in which it could be worn. It was a truly fun day, and we got to know a couple of our fellow travelors well enough to know we would be hanging out and sharing some more outings. But who both Gray and I bonded with the most was Alba Cessani. Alba was to date the most outgoing and vivacious woman, so full of life and love, that I have ever met. And above all, she was sincere. And boy, was she knock out gorgeous.

Before leaving the island, the bartenders, turned us on to some Mexican moonshine called "Raicilla." It is made from the peyote cactus, and has some peyote buttons thrown in for effect. They say not to do more than one or two shots because every batch is different.

As it turned out, along with working at the hotel and modelling, Alba also sold time shares. But when she wasn't working, in the evenings, she would come over and we would all head out together. Everyone in town knew and respected, and above all loved Alba. She knew where to go and when to go, and what was going on everywhere. She got us past all the long line-ups' (because it was Spring Break), and we never had to pay cover charge anywhere. She had me up on podiums dancing, and drinking things out of bottles the staff handed you that made you feel all warm and fuzzy inside. We went to all of the best high end places in Puerto Vallarta with her. We met all of the who's who.

I recall this one night we all went out to one of these outdoor Mexican Fiestas, and since no one knew my name, I wore this awesome white rice material dress that was wonderfully sheer, with only g-strings underneath. There were a lot of pictures taken that night, let me be telling you! Gray loved it. He loved it so much that we went to one of the boutiques that Alba modelled for, and he bought me a g-string bathing suit. It cost a fortune even for Mexico, but it was the coolest bathing suit I had ever seen.

So funny, we were at the beach the next day, and I was wearing my new suit of course. I dozed off face down on the blanket. The next thing I knew Gray was sitting beside me laughing so hard he was crying. When I asked him what had happened, he told me that a local fellow had been walking along the beach and noticed me laying there. Apparently he could not take his eyes off me long enough to see the giant hole some kids had dug in the sand. As he sauntered on he fell head long, right in. Gray figured that entertainment alone paid for the swimsuit.

You know, we had so much fun, that I did not even get a chance to see the roof top swimming pool at our hotel. I think Gray took some pictures of it for me. Before we went home however, we set out on a mission to find us some more of that Raicilla, to bring back home. We smuggled it back in a 60 oz. Vodka bottle, and it was to be reserved for my 30th birthday party. And oh, what a party it turned out to be.

The house that Gray and I occupied was a two storey house, in which Gray had set up a recreation room downstairs. It was complete with the bar (where I first met him), inclusive of full fridge, a snooker pool table (which had the felt replaced once a month) and several pinball machines. There was also a sit down Pac Man table, and a stand up Track and Field machine. You see, one of his sidelines was the rental of pinball and other machines. When he rotated them at the locations, they were rotated through the rec room and entryway as well. As you can well imagine, this meant that we had a lot of company all the time, and of course, most of the parties were held at our place. When I was sick however, we laid low, of course. Everyone in the house was very respectful of me always. My little brother lived there with us for a while, and then Gray's little brother lived there for a while.

So, let me tell you quickly then, about my 30th birthday party Gray threw for me. I recall there were a lot of people. They were milling about everywhere, in the front yard, in the backyard, in the house upstairs, and of course in the house, downstairs. I remember one story Gray had told me about having reached into his clean laundry bag one day, and grasped a handful of puke. Someone had actually vomited in the bag! Whenever Gray threw a party in the past he had made a giant pot of chilli. That was until at one party, I came upstairs, just in time to see a guy whom I had never even seen or met before, lift the ladle complete with chilli to his mouth. Half way back he stopped to puke into the pot, and then kept eating. I had not ever been witness to anything so disgusting and gross in my whole life. That was the last time we made chilli, and especially froze the leftovers!

Back to the party. It was about a week after my initial birthday, because we wanted to have it on the weekend. There had to be about 100 or so people there. Gray, being the stickler that he was, tried to make sure that no one drank too much of the raicilla as he had done in Mexico. So, he had come up with was a plan, that whenever he gave someone a shot (only our closest friends of course) he would mark it on their hand, so no one got more than a couple of shots. He and I had had two shots each before long. I recall meeting him behind the bar and he offered me another shot...I told him that I was feeling pretty wrecked (depending on the batch this stuff could make you hallucinate). I told him to pour me just 1/2 of a shot, and proceeded to drink it. If I am not mistaken, he himself took another two shots himself.

I do not remember how much longer after that it was, but the next thing I recall is looking for Gray and not being able to find him. I went around and around the house and the yard in circles, asking everyone I came across if they had seen Gray. Everyone said "No", they had not run into him. I have no idea how long it was in real time, but it seemed as though I had searched for him for at least two hours, before I finally stumbled upon a white little pickup truck, which for some weird reason was parked in the back yard. As I walked around the truck, I finally found Gray, hanging out of the passenger door, with his head down. "What's the matter?" I asked him. He was green and puking out of the truck door. He had told everyone not to tell me where he was, because I suppose he was embarrassed.

"Well," I told him, "It doesn't bother me, so I'll just hang out here with you." So, between puking we chatted for awhile, I have no idea how long. I ended up crouching in the grass beside the truck. After awhile, I said, "Gray, I need to go pee." "Well go then," he replied. Sure, easy to say, but try as I might, I simply could not move. Really, I could not get up, and it was a really weird sensation. Next thing I know, I had actually started to cry. "I can't get up," I told him. "That's ok, honey," he said, "you're in the grass, you can just pee right there." "Oh, ya," I replied, "what a good idea." And thus, I proceeded to let loose with a pretty big pee. It wasn't until I was done that I realized what had just happened.

You see, I was wearing a white mini skirt, and had completely forgotten to pull it up before I peed. Needless to say, It was now soaked. The next thing I knew, I really broke out in tears. I cried so hard, wondering how I was going to get back into the house without anyone seeing me. I was completely traumatized by this event. And poor Gray, I will never forget...says, "I wish I could help you honey, but...bahhhhhhhblahhhh (barf), I can't!" There was nothing left to do but wait it out, I thought. When we were finally able to move at all, he climbed out of the truck, helped get me to my feet, and we helped carry each other into the house. We had agreed to try to slip past everybody and just go to bed. Just as we thought the coast was clear, and we had made it three quarters of the way up the stairs, in came a slew of new people. One of them I recall being Kurt, the guy that had taken me over here to meet Gray in the first place. We pretty much told them we were messed up and needed to go to bed, but stay and have a good time. So, needless to say, we ended up passed out cold by midnight, and the party went on without us until the next afternoon. Anyone who had had only one or two shots of the moonshine, said they had the best night of their lives. We had obviously done too much.

Now, let's see, what comes next? Oh, yes, the next thing on the agenda would be my best friend's birthday in July of that year. Mandy's birthday, (the girl who's parents took me in the last year of school), is about a month after my own. She and her boyfriend lived in Kelowna at this time, and so we were heading out there for a week long trip. Kelowna is about three and a half hours from Vancouver now, but in those days, before the new highway, it was five hours to get there. It was such a nice drive the old way though, through Yellowstone National Park. Boy, did I ever blow a lot of car speakers driving to and fro all the years Mandy lived there!

I remember that we arrived the day of her actual birthday party. They had a big BBQ and some of their friends were over. Mandy and I had decided we would start by drinking Caesars. Since I had somehow not felt much like drinking lately, Caesars has always been that one standby that I love to sip on when I don't know what to drink. "Strange," I thought, I just couldn't bring myself to drink those either. Mandy asked what was wrong, and I told her that they just were not going down at all. She laughed and made some off handed remark, suggesting that perhaps I was pregnant. I in turn laughed it off. It was a good party anyway though, and we ended up staying for a couple of days.

When we left Mandy's, we headed north-east for another four and a half hours or so, to a town called Golden BC, right on the Alberta/BC border. This was where Gray's sister Wanda lived at the time. For me, it became a most horrible drive. About half way there, I got one of my migraine headaches, and it was a doozy. I got migraines quite often since I was a teenager, and so I always had a migraine preventative on hand. It was a medication called cafergot and is to be taken at the onset of the migraine. Cafergot opens all your sinuses wide, but makes you feel kind of weird. It didn't really work all that well on this trip, because the headache had come on so fast this time, but it did manage to hold it at bay. I think we stayed with Wanda and her husband and their three girl's place for a couple of days, and then began the drive back home. When we arrived back, I immediately made a doctor's appointment, having been feeling kind of weird lately. Also Mandy's prognosis rang in my ears, and I could not shake it.

I will never forget the moment in time a few days later, when Gray pulled up in front of my doctor's office to pick me up. I totally felt as though I were in a daze, in zombie mode, as though I were floating through the air. I must have had a funny look on my face. When he asked me what was wrong with me, I began laughing hysterically, I just didn't know what else to do. I laughed and laughed, until the tears came to my eyes. Finally, he said, "Are you pregnant, by any chance?" I looked over at him, thought to myself, how handsome he was, and suddenly, without warning, I began wailing uncontrollably. I had had no idea how I was going to tell him, and he had made it easier for me. But of course, that was Grayson's style, he made everything easier for me. I know in my heart and in my soul, that had he not come along when he did, I would be dead now, and if not dead, even worse, "the walking dead."

You see, Gray and I had planned to have a child. It was what we both had really, really wanted. It was my number one reason, other than for myself, that I wanted to be clean. I wanted to have a baby more than anything in the world. So, we had mutually decided that I should be clean for one year before getting pregnant, to make sure that the drugs were fully out of my system. Because it seeps right into your bone marrow, the methadone takes a year to completely be released. Having been through what we had been through...my addictions, which often led to very moody and volatile behaviour, and then my long and painful recovery, well...it had been very hard and trying on our relationship, to say the least. Not for one moment, folks, allow yourselves to think that this was ever an easy road for either one of us. In no way would I have blamed him for leaving at any point in time, and I wanted to make sure that he understood that. But, being the man he is, he took the bull by the horns, and plugged through the mire with and for me. Having been through all this stuff had definitely left a lot of scars on our relationship.

I'll tell you guys one story that comes to mind at this moment, that truly depicts the ardour of what I had put the poor guy through. I had quietly, and I thought, inconspicuously wandered into the bedroom, one afternoon, to sneak myself a little bit more dope. To my astonishment and chagrin, my drugs were nowhere in sight. I started to search frantically, and when I looked up, (now having lost all track of time), there he was standing in the doorway, with a sad look on his face. "What have you done," I asked, "where the fuck are my drugs?" "I have them," he said calmly. I told him to give them back, give them back right now. I was truly beginning to panic, not knowing if he had them, or had gotten rid of them. We began arguing profusely, as I tried to find out what he had done with my dope, and he not telling me. "I will give you back your drugs," Gray said, "right after you look at yourself in this mirror," and he pointed to the mirror right in front of me. I started to freak out, I mean I really started to freak out. I felt a violent force boiling up within me. "Give me my fucking dope back, or I will kill you," I screamed. "Just look in the mirror," he stupidly kept repeating. But, I could not. No matter how hard I tried, I could not look at myself like this. I felt myself begin to hyperventilate. I became an animal, right then and there, and a small part of me knew that. That small part of me could not, and would not, no matter what, look at herself in that mirror. It was simply not a possibility. Instead, not knowing what else to do, I lunged at him. Had I gotten a hold of Gray that day, I knew I would most likely have hurt him somehow. Luckily, he got away, and was able to retrieve my dope and throw it back at me, before anything really bad happened. That was the moment in time, that I realized that it is absolutely true what they say, "Never take the dope away from a junkie, that is a bad, bad, idea." In that moment I felt as though I would have killed for my precious dope. I will never, as long as I live, forget what that felt like. It was the worst kind of jail to be in, and it somehow ended up helping me in my own recovery.

Anyways, yes, we had both wanted a baby more than anything else, and spent many days and nights plotting what sort of parents we would be and so on. I had hand picked Grayson Jay Everett Kelly to be the father of my child, for I knew how great of a father and family man he was, and the close knit group his own family represents. Until that moment, there had been no other man that I would have allowed myself to have a child with. As you may remember, I had known Braydon, (Gray's son) since he had just turned 1 year old. I regarded him always as my own, and grew to love this boy oh so very much. Braydon had never been the warm cuddly type, and it was always a very special moment in time (the whole planet would stop) when he took it upon himself to give somebody a hug or a kiss, and if you were that recipient...wow. I saw the same sense of pride and pleasure come across other special people's faces, as I am sure they saw on mine, when Braydon would lean forward for that ever so tentative little peck. Braydon still lives on the island, Vancouver Island, in Victoria, the province's capitol. It was a lot of travel and a lot of time, but we went over there on a ferry every second weekend, to pick him up, and then again on the ferries to bring him back.

It really sucked when Braydon's mom dragged him through the court system, for personal vengeance. For over a year, we travelled back and forth every week. Then, when she convinced the courts that they had to invoke mandatory supervised visitation rights, it became even more difficult. That meant that we had to stay on the island, because the court appointed person was from Victoria. Thank goodness that Gray had family over there, whom we could stay with. Gray kept his cool, though it could not have always been easy, and his whole family supported him throughout, as did I. Grayson would have done whatever it took, until the end of days to be able to see his little boy. It was almost two years later, when Gray finally won "the right" to be with his boy. When Gray was with Braydon, he maintained such a powerful one on one with his son. I always found the bond so very powerful. Gray had a way of always "being in the moment" with us.

This is why there was no doubt in my mind that Grayson would be the best father to my child that I could wish for. We had, however, talked it through, and since we had been arguing more and more lately, we had put off the idea of having a baby at this time. So, I did not know what his response to my being pregnant now would be. Which brings me back to being in the car with him after having just come out of the doctor's office. After I had calmed down a bit, and was no longer laughing hysterically, or crying uncontrollably, we sat in silence for a few minutes. Neither one of us quite knew what to say. When we finally looked at each other, he gently asked if I knew what I intended to do. "I haven't had time to think about it," I said. "Well, I just want you to know that whether you decide to keep the baby, or whether you decide to not keep the baby, it is completely your choice," he said. I appreciated that, but at the same time, of course, I needed to find out what his first choice would be. Needless to say, both of us wanted to keep this baby, and do the best we could.

My pregnancy with Kaytlin was a breeze. I absolutely loved being pregnant. I loved everything about it. I was blessed enough to have any morning sickness, ever, not even once. I felt healthier and more alive than I had ever felt in my life. The timing could not have been better in that I had never been clean before, and having made it 11 months clean, the natural endorphins were beginning to kick in again, and I was once again able to feel that euphoric feeling. I'm not sure if I explained it earlier, but when the body is addicted to an opiate, the natural endorphins (your body's natural opiates) stop being produced, because the opiate is doing the work for the body. I guess what I am trying to get across here is, that I had deadened and dulled my senses for so long with drugs, that when you add the exhilarating feeling of pregnancy and of having a life inside you...well, it is beyond description. It was better than any drugs I had ever taken, that is for certain.

But, you know what they say, nothing is ever perfect. Pregnancy did have some setbacks for me. The main concern was that I had absolutely no sex drive left. The passion I had felt for Gray in the past, which had been so intense, was suddenly gone. I do not know exactly when that happened, if it was even before I got pregnant maybe, but dammit, it happened. Gray happened to be even more highly sexed than I am, and I am basically insatiable when I am in love with someone. But, Gray, well he wanted me all the time, several times a day in fact. I think that what happened to me was that it became a chore, and then, it turned into a kind of resentment. Now, being pregnant gave me an excuse, but as Gray said, he could not last "without' forever. He did warn me several times that he may end up cheating, if I did not have sex with him. But a part of me just could not. The more he wanted it, the more pressure I felt, the more I couldn't bring myself to enjoy it. It completely disappeared for me.

Well, I was about seven months pregnant, when Gray had just come home from working out of town, and we had just gone to bed. I sensed that something was wrong, just before he blurted out that he had something to tell me. I already knew, I told him, because I had already felt it from afar. It was in that moment, as we lay down, and just before he told me, that I knew it to be true. Gray had had a one night stand. Thankfully, he had been smart enough, and sensitive enough, I suppose (in hindsight), to have made sure that it was not someone he would ever see again. But it hurt me to the quick, and of course it did not make anything that we were going through any easier. Shit, another cloud hanging over our heads. And, honestly, I could seriously not blame him for having done it. I suppose that if I were the recipient of rejection, I may even have done the same. Although I have never, ever cheated on any man that I have ever been in a serious committed relationship with. Not even when I thought they would deserve it.

So, from there things progressed, as my tummy grew. I have to tell you though, that even at five and six months pregnant, you could not really tell. I carried my baby straight out and quite high. My favourite story of pregnancy is about to be told here. Bet you could already feel it, hey? I had been going to "narcotics anonymous" meetings regularly since I was well enough to attend. The meetings, I later discovered were another form of addiction to a lot of its' members. I met people that consistently booked off from work to attend a meeting. It became their main focus, and in my opinion, there were members that used the meetings as their new drug. I, however, did not get that deeply involved.

There was a fellow there though, whom I had befriended, and he was really nice and really cute. He used to phone me at home to see how I was doing, and I think it kind of made Gray jealous. Anyway, my best friend was a stripper (dancer), and had been since she was just out of school at eighteen. She had a dancing gig at a local bar, and wanted me to come along and hang out with her, which I did on occasion. I was sitting at a bar in the upper section where the dancers and staff sat, sipping on my virgin Caesar, when I caught sight of the guy from my meetings. He sat down with a friend right in front of me, actually. We were both surprised to see each other there, and I don't know what was in his drink, but I was quick to assure him that mine was non alcoholic. It needs to be stated here that most drug addicts cannot partake in drinking alcohol, because nine times out of ten, it leads them back to their drug of choice. I am most fortunate not to be in that category. I have always been able to drink socially, and not want the drugs because of it. More than likely, now that I have analyzed this, I think it is because I do not drink in excess. I have always felt nauseous if I had one too many drinks, and would automatically slow down or stop drinking all together. I was known amongst my friends to "nurse" my drinks, and it seemed to bother them sometimes.

Back to my favourite tale though...they were in the bar that afternoon in question. A few of the Budweiser girls, and they had gone up on stage and performed a few gyrating dances. After they were done, they hung out at the club for a couple of hours, getting to know the customers and signing autographs. Well, it was really weird, but before I knew what was happening, I was surrounded by a bunch of guys, who apparently thought that I was a Budweiser girl! Here I was sitting there, five months pregnant, drinking virgin cocktails, and minding my own business. I laughed and told them all that I was not a Budweiser girl, and although I was flattered, I could therefore not sign any autographs for them. Well, do you think that these poor sods would believe me? The more I denied it, the more they stuck their pens and paper in my face, begging for my signature. So, needless to say, what was a girl to do? I started signing autographs. I had so much fun that day, I cannot even tell you. I signed so many autographs that I started to feel like a celebrity.

I think that it was a total drain on me knowing that Gray had cheated on me, and that he was consistently working out of town. I will never forget this one afternoon, when we were both standing in the bedroom in front of the tall dresser, and we were having a heated argument. I do not recall what it was even about, but it was one of those doozies, and it was loud. We were both screaming at each other, and before I knew what had happened, I saw him lift his hand and, then it connected with my head. We had argued a lot before, but he had never actually hit me. Not until that day. I was eight months "along" at the time.

I was stunned, completely stunned. I did not know what to do, or how to handle this one. I believe I ran out of there, hopped into the car, and drove somewhere. I do not remember where I drove. I know however, that I called my little brother and told him that Gray had just hit me. He was irate, but I did not know how mad he was, until later that day, when there was a knock at the door. There he stood, a nose away from Gray, demanding that he step outside. Now, I have never seen my brother hit anyone before, or even get in a position where I thought he might. Matt has always been the peace keeper in my family. Boy, oh boy, he was mad. Gray and he ended up talking it out instead, and Matt came in and made sure that I was ok, before he let it go. It wasn't until that moment that I knew that he would always do anything to protect me, my little brother, and I felt a wave of love for him, that was so powerful.

Needless to say, I do not think that things were ever the same again after that between Gray and I. There was just too much damage done. As the time grew closer to my having the baby, I wanted this thing out of me more than anything else in the world. Every morning near the end that I awoke and still had the giant belly, I was angry. I thought that it would happen like it does in the movies, and that I would wake up in the middle of the night with contractions, and be raced to the hospital. Well, not quite. The coolest thing I remember though, and at the time I had no idea who it was doing it, (and that made it even better and more intriguing) was that every morning I got up, I would look outside our living room window, and sure enough (for at least two weeks every single morning), there it would be. Unbeknownst to us at the time, my brother and sister in law, who had just had a baby themselves, had made a stork. They pierced into the lawn in front of the door of our house, and every morning without fail there would be new baby gifts in the stork's beak. Little rattles, and bibs, and well, you get the picture? Every morning, it would dispel my anger for not having had my baby during the night.

It turned out that I had now made it two weeks to the day past my due date, and I was frantic to get rid of this thing inside me. I ended up at an ultrasound appointment to see if they were going to need to do something or not. To my surprise, they nurses told me that I was in labour, as in right now, I was in labour! I could not believe it, I was so excited. I, however could not understand that if I was indeed in labour, why was I not also in pain? I called Gray and told him the news. Then I raced home, made sure that everything I needed was packed, and out we headed. Knowing that they were not going to let me eat at the hospital, he decided to take me out for breakfast first. I still have the pictures of us leaving the house that day. Too funny...there I am, in a purple jumpsuit, posing all sassy like in profile view, getting into Gray's bright yellow little pick up truck. I remember thinking, "Boy, this is going to be a lot easier than I thought." So, off to some restaurant in our neighbourhood, we headed, and of course, Gray had to go and tell our waitress that I was in labour. He freaked out the poor girl, who was scared to serve us, and asked should we not be at the hospital instead. She was truly terrified, I think. But serve us she did.

Then we left and headed for the hospital, were calmly admitted, and again I thought to myself, "This is not how I thought it would be, not at all the way I had seen it time and again on television." Believe me when I say that it got a lot harder. There was another woman in my semi private room, who as I recall was 41 years old and being in great shape. She spit her baby out within two hours of arrival. Not me! I ended up in intense pain for the next twenty four and a half hours. They gave me an epidural and it did not work. The shot, which is given in your spine is supposed to freeze you from the waist down. In my case, however, it only froze my left leg. The second shot, for which I had to beg, was not any better. I was told that the epidural shots do not work for everybody. I dilated up to seven centimetres and did not dilate further. Apparently, one has to be ten centimetres dilated to give birth. My baby had been turned "sunny side up", and in order clear the birth canal they have to be facing downwards. They were just about to induce labour, having wheeled the intravenous pole right up beside me, when she decided to turn. I was so grateful for that, because the nurses had mentioned that when one is induced, the pain goes up tenfold, and that I could hardly imagine.

Gray was in the delivery room with me, and finally, out she came. You cannot imagine my surprise that the baby was a girl. I had wanted to have a girl in the worst way possible, more even than a boy, although I would have loved him just the same, I am sure. You see, when I was about five or six months along, Gray and I had gone to an ultrasound appointment together and both of us thought we saw huge balls, and a penis. Well, we told everyone who would listen that we were having a boy. At that time, doctors were allowed to determine whether their patients were told the sex of the fetes or not, and mine did not, nor would I have wanted to know for sure first.

There had been two baby showers thrown for me, and everything we were given was geared towards us having a boy. Lots of blue things, for sure. Kaytlin Diana Kelly came into this shining world a whopping 6 lb, 9 ounces, which, it turned out was a good birth weight. My doctor had been worried throughout my pregnancy that the baby might be low birth weight, because I was so small. Kaytlin had made up for lost time in the end that is for sure. The moment she was born, I discovered a new sort of love. I suppose that there is absolutely no way in this universe to adequately describe the feelings that I felt when my darling daughter was born. It was by far the best thing that had ever happened to me. I was completely overwhelmed.

I will never forget the ride home from a hospital a couple of days later. We had been given so many clothes for our newborn infant, but she swam in everything. We finally settled on a little green outfit, that consisted of pants with closed feet, and a sweater to match. It was the tiniest thing we had, and it was still too large. When we got out to the car, Gray had to strap her into the car seat in the back, which I hated because I did not want to let go of her. I remember so clearly now, turning around in my passenger seat, and staring at this tiny little stranger in the back. I do not know what overcame me, but suddenly I began to cry uncontrollably. I cried like I had never cried before. I cried and I cried, and I cried, all the way home. Gray did not say much, I think that he understood somehow that this was the biggest, most real thing that had ever happened to me.

Grayson Jay Everett Valentine Kelly was a huge help to me when we got home with Kaytlin. He had taken some time off work, to help me out. I do not know if I have mentioned this before, but when I first met him, he drove a dump truck and worked together with his father. He hated the business. He had done the same thing for far too long now, and wanted out. They dealt mainly with lime and mushroom manure type hauls.

We started looking for something else that he wanted to do for a living, and after some research, he ran across something that is called non-destructive testing. It wasn't long after that, that he sent away for the materials and began the course. A couple of his friends were in the business, and so he would come out of it with a job. Now, what "NDT testing" is, is this. They use different forms of testing, but mainly they use radiation testing, to test things like bridges, air planes, and tanks, for cracks or weak spots. They have devices that measure how much radiation they are subjected to on every job, as they hide behind lead shields. It is an extremely dangerous job, because as we all know, radiation, if one gets in contact with it, will burn a human being from the inside out. I never did like that he had chosen this risky career, but the pay obviously was really good, and he loved it. Another down side to all this, a huge down side was that he was out of town all the time, because they had to test tanks and equipment when the mills were on shut down, all over Canada. Gray had begun this career before Kaytlin was born, and now he was getting called out more and more often.

After we had gotten our daughter home, I was so scared to handle her. I did not realize it, but I knew nothing about babies. I used to babysit when I was younger, but they were not new borne, and I'd maybe changed a diaper once or twice and plucked a bottle in some babies' mouth, a couple of times perhaps, for I could not even remember it really. I was so scared that I might break this delicate little bundle. The first few times we had to give Kaytlin a bath, Gray had to do it, for I was certain that she would slip out of my soapy hands, and end up drowning. Gray was so patient with me though, and helped me to get the confidence I needed. My sister in law had just had a baby herself two months prior, so she encouraged me as well. To this very day, her daughter Lauren and my daughter have remained close. They were always together growing up.

Well, it wasn't long at all, before he had to go back to work. But again, I was really lucky. When I was about seven months pregnant, some friends of Gray's, a married couple by the names of Carmen and Will, whom I really liked, had some company from out of country. Carmen's sister Sharlene had come to visit them from Melbourne, Australia. Carmen, herself was pregnant and our kids ended up being born two months apart as well. She later had another boy who is one year younger than Kaytlin, and the three of them also grew up together.

The evening I met Sharlene we all had so much fun. You know, every once in a while, as we walk through this life, we meet somehow whom we have that automatic connection with? The sort of person whom, if you do not see them for twenty years, it will be as though no time has passed. Sharlene was my soul mate to be sure. After that evening she and I saw a lot of each other, and as soon as Gray zipped out of town, she was staying at our place, rather than her sister's. As a matter of fact, Sharlene remained with us until Kaytlin was five months old. Her visa had expired, and she had no choice but to go back to Australia. Sharlene helped me to raise my daughter for the first five months of her little life, and she was an unbelievable, and most welcome guest. She ended up coming back when KK (which Gray and I have always lovingly called her) was one year old, until she was almost two. She lived with us for a couple of those months, but then began dating a friend of mine and Gray's, and ended up staying mostly with him.

Now, I'm not sure if you recall my telling you earlier, that Gray and I had not been getting along very well, even before my pregnancy, which is why we had decided to put it off. After Kaytlin was born, it seemed to escalate, and we found ourselves fighting all the time. It was awful. One thing that made things so difficult was the fact the Gray worked out of town so much. I understand now that it is very difficult on any relationship. You live a certain life style, and you see different people, and you plan your days and nights differently, than when the other party suddenly blitzes back in through the front door. All of a sudden, I had to adapt again to a totally different life style where my focus was supposed to be around him. It is so hard when you are in this sort of scenario, almost like an on and off switch. By the time I would get comfortable having Gray home again, he would be leaving.

Since all I ever heard when I was growing up, was my parents fighting, and knowing what a negative impact that can have on the rest of your life, I wanted to break the cycle. I wanted to break the cycle my parent had raised me in, in every way humanly possible. I did not ever want to parent my daughter the same way that I had been raised. The most important thing to me then and now, was that I raise my daughter to be strong, self sufficient, and most of all confident. I do not think that there has ever been a day that has gone by that I have not told my daughter that I love her. My parents never, ever told me that they loved me, they never, ever, told me that they were proud of me. They never, ever, kissed me, or hugged me, not that I can recall. The putdowns, and the negative affirmations however, were second nature for them. I suppose they had their own crosses to bear, and maybe they have done the best they can, with the tools that they were given. I still feel in my heart though, that my mom and dad, were two individuals who should never have had children. My parents care only about their owns lives, and their own feelings. They cannot seem to be able to feel the feelings of the ones they love. I still hate the thought that maybe they seriously just do not care. My mother especially, (for I feel it in my heart) does not like me.

So, having been a part of all the fighting and screaming in my house, I did not want a child of mine to go through the same daily stress, and that is what had become of Gray's and my relationship. So, it was time to have "the talk." We both amicably agreed that this not working out, and that I was going to leave him in the house he already had before I came along. Kaytlin, then five months old, and I, would move out. It was extremely difficult for me, because I was still totally in love with Gray at the time. I think that most of you out there know how difficult it can be to throw in the towel when you are still in love, through and through. But I did it for my daughter, and we all know, that it would just be a matter of time anyway.

And, so, I went out and found us a quaint little two bedroom basement suite in the same city. It, still to this day, is the place that Kaytlin and I remember the most fondly. Even though she was so young, she remembers it quite well. We lived in that suite until Kaytlin was almost five years old, and I hate to admit, it was to be the longest lasting residence, up until this very date. The house was very new, and clean and bright. The kitchen was large and with the sliding glass doors, into the back yard and the patio, drew in a lot of light. In the living room there was another window. I don't know why, but natural sunlight in my home is the most important aspect for me. I hated that Gray had always had the curtains drawn in our place. He liked it dark and dingy. Kaytlin and I actually thrived in this place. There was a super nice family upstairs and they had three daughters of their own.

Looking back upon on that time now, I just realized at this very moment, that the five years after I had left Gray were the best of my life. I completely forgot to tell you earlier that when I was still with him, and other than the times that I had spent in detox and six months recuperating, I had been working steadily, of course. I worked at Revenue Canada Taxation when I met Gray. Now, that is where I ended up applying after I had worked downtown at Block Bros. Head Office, if you recall. It was the year of Expo Vancouver 1986, when I had lost my job at Block Bros. and got another at taxation. The money was pretty good for the 80's, and I always had plenty in my bank account. After all, I was on the methadone program, so it wasn't all being spent on dope. Thank Gosh that taxation was only a seasonal job, because it was bar none the most hated and boring job I had ever done. I worked in data entry, and they had three different pay levels, based on your speed. It took me a couple of years to get to Level 3, but then I was able to maintain it.

Anyways, while I was still with Gray, I went back to night school and took conveyance. I had done conveyance, but from a different angle at Block Bros head office. It was a real estate conveyance, which is basically the paper work that real estates handle in the transfer of a property. The course I took though, was law firm conveyancing. I was a legal conveyance secretary, and what we essentially did was to draw up all the legal paperwork for one of the parties in a real estate transaction. This led to the transfer of the property in question at Land Title office on a certain day by a certain time, usually the 15 and the 30th or 31st of every month. Conveyance is one of the most high pressure jobs in the world when the market is hot, and at that time it certainly was. There was no time to look at the clock, and I loved the job and the pressure. At the first law firm I worked at, I also learned that doctors and lawyers were about to no longer intimidate me. The man I worked for was a lazy, pompous, sloppy child. We did all the work for him. We even ended up with the wills and estates files, when irate clients came raging into the office demanding their paperwork.

I had initially been hired on for three months as a temp, while his conveyor was off on maternity leave. Three or four weeks before my time was to expire, I of course went out to seek other employment. I had even told him that I was looking, so I could use him as a referral. The next thing I knew, I was offered a really great position with a neighbouring notary public, and she had offered to pay me a full $2,000 more per month than I was getting paid. I must admit that the reason for that was, that when she asked me what I made now, I mistakenly wrote down the wrong figure. When I told him who it was that had offered me a job, he was not happy, not happy at all. It turned out they had been partners a few years prior, and he decided that he was now going to keep me, rather than let her have me.

The only thing was that, he didn't have the balls to tell me this himself, or to offer me more money. Instead, he called her and threatened to black ball her in the business, and apparently he could have. The next thing I knew, she phoned me and told me that it had just been found out that she had a terminal illness, and would now have to be laid up for a while. She explained that she would have to put her business on hold. It turned out that this was total bullshit, a story they had concocted up together. He ended up calling me out to have a smoke with him at work, and went on about how terrible it was that she had "aids." I later found out that none of it was true. I then called Stan into his own office, whereupon, I called him a "parasitic ditch pig," and any other name that popped to mind, and then threw him back out of his own office. Slamming the door after him, I told him that I quit. That was fun! Good thing I had a third job already lined up!

It was somewhat of a shame, because as I was saying, I did not want anyone else to raise my daughter. Someone had told me once that the first five years of a child's life are the most formative years. It is said that we learn more in the first five years than in the rest of our entire lives. It was so important for me to instil my own values in my child. So, when Kaytlin was born, I gave up my job, although I was very happy at another law office, with a great employer. And so I went back to Revenue Canada.

But, I have to say, Petra Hoffmann always gets bored easily, and doing one or two things at a time, has never been enough to keep me stimulated. So, I made another decision. I would also go back to school. This time, I had decided that I would try my hand at Real Estate. It was to be a six month correspondence program, if you gave it at least five hours a day. And believe me when I say, you cannot cheat yourself of those hours. Sixty-eight percent fail the test the first time through, and there are only three chances. If you have to take it a second time, you have to wait another three months, and pay for the next exam. If you fail that one, you have to wait another year to try a third time.

Alright, so where does that put me now? Let me give you my schedule as I recall it, say from January on, when I would have started back at Revenue Canada. Kaytlin would have been ten months old. My shift at work would start at 3:30 pm. I had to drive Kaytlin to my mother in law's house, at about 2:30. I would get off of work at 11:30 pm, drive back to my mother and father in law's, pick up KK, who would be sleeping, while I strapped her in and out of the car seat. I would get home at about 12 or 12:30, tuck in my warm little bundle, and then study until my eyes would fall shut.

I was lucky that KK would sleep in until about 10 am. Sometimes, if I was able, I would try to get up earlier, because it was really hard to study in the mornings with all the distractions and needs of a toddler. It was not easy, but I still tried to find time on the weekends to go out at least one night with my friends, to unwind, and get some "mommy time." Gray would usually take KK then. I have to tell you that I have always been very lucky in that I have never had to leave my daughter with a stranger. If I could not get family or friends to baby sit, I would forfeit going out. Allow me to tell you at this point, that my mother and father in law have always been there for me and KK, in every capacity. It was a crazy busy time, but I loved it. The only part that I found really stressful, and truly did not like, was trying to get out of the house with a toddler. I was always racing the clock. I try not to do that anymore...race the clock...it is so unhealthy.

I sure did study hard, though, and I was able to attend some evening classes, after my few months employ at taxation were over. And, so, in 1992, after Kayla had turned one year old, I ended up at the Pan Pacific Hotel in downtown Vancouver to take my Real Estate exam. It really was a big deal, there were about 300 pupils writing that day. I was so completely nervous. I can honestly say that I had never been so nervous to write a test in my whole life. There were a few of us sitting outside, have a smoke while we waited, and there was a girl there that noticed my discomfort. We began chatting, and she finally convinced me to take this pill to calm me down, some herbal remedy. I don't know why I trusted her, but I checked out the bottle, from a health food store, and I took this little pill.

Sure enough, it calmed me down so much, that I was one of the first people to finish the test, and that just never happens. I am such a slow poke, and am usually one of the last to finish anything. I was told that it is because I was born left handed. In Germany, it was illegal to write left handed in school, and so they taught me how to write right handed. I have seen shows and read studies, and apparently, it is different sides of the brain that send and receive signals when a person is left handed. When they change that, the message has to be resent, and there is a lapse, that slows us down. So, basically, I am slow at everything I do, and confused as to being left or right handed. It is so funny, because, in baseball, for example, I hit the ball right handed, I catch the ball left handed, then I have to throw down the glove in order to throw the ball left handed as well. Generally, I do not pay attention to whether I use my right or left hand, but just tend to do things naturally.

So the day I took my real estate exam was an extremely surreal sort of day. It was warm and sunny in beautiful Vancouver that day. I remember as I left the testing room, and then walked outside, that "knowing" feeling in my heart and in my soul that I had passed. I felt it in every fibre of my being, beyond a shadow of a doubt, and for some strange reason all I could think about was to call my dad, and to share this great I recall telling you earlier about the time I called my dad when he told me how truly proud he was of me. I nearly brought me to my knees, for I really felt that he had not just said the words, he had actually felt them.

After I had hung up the phone, a few more students came towards me, and we had planned to go for a celebration lunch afterwards. As we all started walking down the sidewalk together, I felt charmed. It was a very strange day, as I had mentioned a moment ago, and the next thing I knew, a really nice jaguar pulled up beside us. The driver leaned over to look at me, and to ask for directions to somewhere. "Wait a minute," I thought to myself, "I know this guy!" "Stuart! Stuart McMann, isn't it?" I exclaimed. And, sure enough, it was. I had not seen him since high school, but he was a super popular guy I went to school with, and all the girls had had a crush on him. I quickly told him why and where we were all going and to please come and join us for a drink. I'm not sure why this all stands out in my mind so much, other than that, years ago, in school, he would not have paid me the time of day. Anyway, it ended up being one of the best days and the best lunches, I have ever had. It just felt so good to be alive, and I felt such a rare sense of accomplishment.

# Chapter 5 - Me and Ralph

So then, without further ado, this brings us right up to July 1992. Jeez, guys, looking back, wouldn't you know it! That was at exactly the same time that the Real Estate market took a huge dive! The entire economy took a little dip...we hit a giant friggin' black hole, ladies and gentlemen, boys and girls. Yuppydoodles... the luck of the Hoffmann's. Cannot seem to shake it, not yet, but I am still working wholeheartedly every day, on changing my thinking and therefore, hopefully, my luck. Although I struggled at real estate without a penny to my name, I sure made up for it in fun. I obviously met a whole new array of people, and if you were to ask any of my longstanding friends, they would tell you that 1992/93 were the best years of my life. No one had ever seen me happier.

Sure, I sold a few homes, but the industry is very difficult to break into without money to invest. Very few make it to the top (the top 1% making 95% of all of the money), but when you enter the business at the beginning of a recession, without a pot to piss in, well, my dreams of success and prosperity soon went out the window.

So, what was a girl to do? I am not sure if I had mentioned it, but after having been split up with Gray for a year, we had tried again to make us work. We lasted two months. You see, although I still love the man dearly to this very day, I had fallen "out of love" with him by this point. The chemistry and the magic we once shared were not to return. From what my family on both sides and some of my closest friends have told me, Grayson had really wanted to marry me, and was still also totally in love with me. He told my mother once that I had ruined his life. If I recall in my foggy head correctly, he had told his mother and my sister in law the same thing. It was another guilt that I had to live with.

Well, the year after Gray and I had valiantly tried again, was actually one of the best years I had ever had. I had been raised with weird beliefs surrounding sex, as I may have mentioned earlier. It had been Gray that taught me to get over my own inhibitions. He had truly set me free...free enough to throw all caution to the wind that next year, and to allow myself to do whatever I wanted and to be me. I ended up meeting and seeing three different men. And, boy...were they different. One of them, (you guessed it) was a realtor. He had dealt for many years and was quite well off financially. He took me to all of the nice places. Cory totally wined and dined me, and the best part was that he also had a really nice boat. There is, for me, no better place on earth than on the ocean. I hate being in the water, but I love to be on it. The ocean is the only place where I always find hat inner peace we all struggle so hard to find. I find it there every time, no matter how bad things are, all my worries dissipate. It's almost as good as drugs.

Anyways, Cory was the one who took me to all the nicest places, and he was a lot of fun to be around and hang out with. Neither one of us had any expectations except to have fun. And he was extremely sexual, and the part I loved...creative. Myself, I have found that it is to this day very difficult for me to make the first moves. My fear of rejection is still so strong. I love it when a man takes full charge, and I can lose myself in it. We did things I had never done, (not sexually) but where and when. So, then, I will leave you with one more story about Cory and I...it is one of my favourite to date. You know, for all the misery and hardship I have endured, and for however difficult my life has been, I sure have had a lot of fun and good times, and great memories along the way. My life has certainly been full, "Never a dull moment in Petra World, I always say." I suppose that having grown up so shy, I was now doing exactly the opposite, and maybe even at times have taken it too far. I have yet to find the balance, and am working on it everyday.

Anyways, Cory and I had had an open house in a subdivision we shared, in one of the newest up and coming high end neighbourhoods. After our open, we decided to go to the pub for a drink, which was always a bit risky for me, and I will tell you why later. We stayed for a couple of hours, and then got in his car to go for a drive downtown. There we ended up in Stanley Park, Vancouver's biggest park. Oh, yes, we had gone somewhere fancy for dinner first, but I can't remember where? Anyways, we ended up in the park to witness a beautiful sunset over the ocean. Just before it began to get dark, we had moved our spot into the thicker woods, and laid out a blanket. I had brought some candles, and we cracked open a bottle of wine. We were set...always ready for anything, him and I. After we made love right there in Stanley Park, we fell asleep barely clothed. Well...the next thing I know, I hear this really loud whizzing noise right beside my head. It was so close that I could feel a breeze from the direction of the noise. I looked up, blinded by the light, to see another one coming towards me. We had fallen asleep right beside the main bike trail, and there were cyclists whizzing right by us, barely missing us, for goodness sakes.

Groggy, tired and hung over, we gathered up our stuff, and headed back to the bar to pick up my car which I had left there. As we pulled up in front, on this beautiful, sunny, hot summer day... Cory started killing himself laughing. He laughed so hard he cried, for Gosh's sakes. I looked down at my clothes and realized that I was in very high heels, and my burgundy red leather skirt, and it was obvious that these were the clothes on a girl that she "had worn the night before." So, you can only imagine what was going through my head as I heard his laughter. As I looked over to the right, it slowly dawned on me that the pub was having their annual Car Show. Oops...there mine sat, right in the middle of all the chaos.

Now, any other day, I would have said, "Keep driving, Mister," but I could not, for you see, I had another open house I had to be at in an hour. Dear Gosh, Cory laughed even harder, if that was possible, as I slowly and painstakingly got out of his fancy car, with everybody watching. With my head held high, I climbed up the hill of the steep driveway, found my car amidst all those beauties. Then I politely asked the folks in charge if they could please move like about four vehicles, so that I could get out. The last thing I remember, was Cory's face, still sitting and laughing in his car, and waving, as I slowly pulled out of the driveway, some time later. Had to see it all, he did. What a show, alright! Haha

Oh, yes, how could I forget? I lied when I said that that was the last Cory story I wanted to tell you guys. This one, cannot go without the telling. Somehow, it was one of the most freeing experiencing of entire life. Being the small world that it is we live in, we discovered that Cory had also lived in my home town, and gone to the same high school as I had. We got to talking about it one night, and it turned out that his best friend then, and to this day was a fellow whom I remembered quite well from school. We decided to go out on the boat one night and Cory invited Darren along. It was a perfect summer evening on the ocean, and as the sun began to set in one of the most awe striking ocean sunsets, we pulled up the rest of the crab in our nets. Cory, being the romantic that he was, brought out the champagne, strawberries, and guess what, the whipping cream. After sprinting up to the bridge, where they both had me in turn, we ended back downstairs, laughing, exuberant and oh, so very happy. We were literally high on life.

Well, almost...the next thing I recall was leaning over the table to feed Darren a strawberry as I had been "told" to do. Just as he started playing with my breasts, I felt a very solid presence behind me. "Sublime...just simply sublime," was what went through my mind. That was just before the table broke, and we all lay in a heap on one of the benches. Now, some of you, (and I feel bad for my daughter who may be reading this) may think of me as quite the slut, but ask me if I care? I would not have given up that particular experience for all the tea in China. In fact, we have laughed and giggled about it many times since. As we were leaving the boat that night, I actually fell to my knees, hugged them both around the legs. I thanked them profusely, as I had never thanked anyone before, for one of "the most incredible experiences of my life!"

I am beginning to believe that in those moments, when we experience the world and each other so fully, that we become closer to Gosh, and to all that makes up the Universe. Cory was a ton of fun, for sure, but I had actually made another friend as well. It had been the first time that a girlfriend had taken me to what later turned out to be my favourite pub. We sat on an outdoor patio, and when you walked inside you went down a couple of steps, and there was a lower level. Well, every time I had to go to the washroom, I had to go by a table of three men, who were definitely aware of us there, and wanted nothing more than to meet us. There were actually pretty hilarious and made a lot of funny comments and invited us every time we passed. Then, before I knew it, for we had not been there for very long, Darla rose up and said that she had to leave. I was in no mood to go home yet, and opted to stay by myself. Sure, I knew of course that I would not be alone for long.

It took maybe a minute and two before a couple of them were sitting at my table, to invite me to theirs. And so, I merrily followed them inside. One of the guys was a super tall gangly guy named Dan. He was one of the funniest people I have ever met. He somehow reminds me of "Kramer." The other two guys were brothers, it turned out. One was big and had a big beer belly, biker look, and the other was the opposite in stature, very small, and wiry. He was the one who owned a Harley. Both were very cute and charismatic. And, you know, (as much as us girls all hate this part)...they were actually arguing over who should be with me. Long story short, we left there, and were to meet at a restaurant in a neighbouring town. Only thing was that Jack wanted to show off his bike, and invited me to go with him to the beach. I was wearing a dress, so I declined.

Ralph, his brother suggested that we meet him there. Dan, Ralph and I climbed into his truck as Jack zoomed off, only Ralph had had no intention of following him. We went straight to the restaurant, where he got a jump start on his brother in getting to know me better. Jack finally showed up, and was obviously pissed off. Although he was the better looking of the two by far, there was something about Ralph that I was drawn to. I don't trust people who need to show off and perhaps that is why I chose Ralph over Jack that night.

Needless to say, I ended up at Ralph Raker's place that night, and pretty much from then onward. Ralph was the fun, impromptu, spur of the moment piss tank, life of the party kind of guy. He had his own small business when we met, and had a big house by himself, having just split up with the "love of his life" who had left him and married his best friend. Ralph was a mess, and like a child, he cried bitterly over his loss and drank from morning until night. It was so bad, that he was puking blood in the mornings. I kind of kept him around to party with, and to go trucking with. We went to nightclubs, and had a lot of stripper bar kind of fun. Physically it was the best chemistry I had ever known with a man. It was uninhibited, four/five times a day sex, everywhere and anywhere, and soft and hard, and sultry and exciting. That was what drew me to him, not his whining or the fact that I would want anything more from him than that.

And...ladies and gentlemen, without further ado. Yes...drum roll please...allow me to introduce to you gentleman number three (haha). Micky Pollo was anything but a gentleman. But, again, fun... fun...and very exciting sex. Micky had a house overlooking the ocean, where we would wake up in the living room on a mattress we had tossed there the night before. Micky was the one I would go to visit (aka...booty call) at 5 o'clock in the morning, and he would always open the door. Micky and I did a lot of blow together, and we would stay up all night having crazy wild sex. It really was the best year of my entire life in as much fun that I had, the places I was taken, and the things I did and experienced. I had never felt so free.

But, alas, all good things always come to an end sooner or later, don't they? Now, let me be clear here. I had never led any of them on, they knew that I had come out of a relationship and just wanted to have fun. Work hard, play hard...you know? And along came the spider (I mean the crab), you know the Cancer sign trait... crawling sideways like a crab? Along came Ralph. All three knew that I was seeing three men, and that they were not the only ones, and everyone was ok with it. It got a bit tricky sometimes, because we all hung out at the same bar. Well, not Micky, he had done his time there, as he had been involved for many years prior, with the bartender. It had been a long torrid relationship for them both, so he didn't go there much.

Anyways, Ralph decided one day, I guess, that he now wanted me all for himself, and began hanging out so much, that I soon had no time for the others. They just kind of gradually faded into the distance. And with that began another interesting era in the life and times of Petra Hoffmann!

Kaytlin would have been four years old at this point, so I had actually been alone for a while. We still lived in our favourite basement suite, the first one we lived at since Gray, where she had learned to walk, and she had learned to talk, and to fall and to crawl, and to cry, scream, laugh, and play. Gray, during this span, had been taking her most weekends so that I could work and play. Real Estate, however had been really tough. The market, as I explained earlier had crashed and we had hit a recession. I had no more money to throw after the bad, and was now working with a less expensive office. Actually, Cory had ended up there also. I can't remember who went there first, him I think.

Me, I started to stay over at Ralph's more and more, when KK was at Gray's or his parents' place. They were all so great, the Kelly family. I was the luckiest single parent I knew in that they were always there for us both, through thick and thin. Real estate was definitely more difficult than a eight hour a day job, like taxation had been. When one works selling houses, you often get a call, and have to drop whatever you are doing. Like a showing that night, say at 8pm, when people are home from work, and after they have had dinner. The hours made it impossible, for I could not just drop everything and leave KK and it cost me more than a few sales to be sure.

Ralph did not meet my daughter until we had been seeing one another for a year. Until then I had not had anyone around other than Micky once in a while, when she was home. She hated any guy she had ever felt that I had chemistry with. Kaytlin has always been extremely demanding of attention, and looking back that is probably one of my biggest mistakes in parenting. I had a lot of friends, and they were around a lot, when I could not go out. I have always been very much a "people person," and very outgoing, oftentimes paying more attention to my friends than to KK.

So, Ralph had a two story house, and within two more months time, had convinced me to move in with him. I really thought I loved this man, and agreed that if we got a new place, I would love to move in together. So, I gave up my suite that we loved so much, my "baby dolly" and I. Baby Dolly is the pet name that Gray gave to our daughter. Ralph gave up his house, and fucking...ouch... somehow his job disintegrated! Hello!!! Had I NOT been through this before? Red flag, red flag, another red flag...like the alcoholism was not enough. And what do we tell ourselves ladies? "He's just drinking so much, because he is so sensitive and has a broken heart. Since he is so sensitive it makes me love him even more. He loves me now and my love can fix him." In fact, after all I had been through, it embarrasses me so much now to have to tell you about how bad this relationship became. I confused (once again), love and lust, I put up with the stupidest things. Things I could never believe others should put up with. So, I ask you, which is the one that is really blind? Love or Lust. I call lust...it has hurt me more in my life than love ever has.

I hardly know where to begin. Other than the drinking, he also smoked weed from morning until night. It would be rolled on his bedside table in the morning. Because he had been self employed and his partner had fallen completely under the hell gates of crack, Ralph ended up on social assistance. This was not enough to cover even his half of the rent, and I had to cover that. But who do you think bought the groceries, put gas in the cars, and who do you think, began drinking more than ever, and I ended up buying his beer too? If you can't beat them, join them, was the defeatist attitude I obviously had. So figure it out...he had talked me into a nice house in Panorama Ridge, which was in a high end subdivision, and I was a single mother, just starting a new business in real estate without any money. I was fucked.

Yes, but that was not enough for Petra, see, it gets worse, a lot worse. So many stories, that at least it was never ever boring. The long and short of it was, that he could not keep his pecker in his pants for more than a few hours. And, yes, I thought that I would ignore that too. In fact, two of his "friends" would come over to MY house and hang out in the shop with him, and leave me all alone in the house. If I did join them, it felt so uncomfortable and stifled, I was sure that they were actually laughing at me, and they were. They were also ten years his junior.

Ralph had me so controlled and manipulated ( I used to call him the Master Manipulator) and I found out later, that I was not the only one of course. I was actually afraid to go down to his shop, my heart would pound the whole way, and then feeling shunned, it was not worth the effort to keep an eye on him. One day, for example, I had just driven out of the driveway to go to work, and got only half block away, before I turned around, for I had forgotten something. Damn, her car was already there, she had to have been at the end of the block waiting for me to pull out, there could be no other explanation. Again...nothing but lies and deceit...and me choosing to believe the lies. See, for the three and a half years that I was with Ralph, our sexual relationship got better and better, and I had never even heard of that. We always found a way to make it new and different, and exciting in bed. I realize now that was the only reason I stayed. I still miss the uninhibited way in which we made love...Gray had given me wings to fly uninhibited, and Ralph had then become the most exciting lover I had ever known. He was a total sex addict, and so it was always exciting and he loved to do the work, if you know what I mean.

I have just had a recollection that I must throw in here, although it may be a bit out of context. It is basically about this girl whom I had met once, a few months earlier. Cory (boat-dude) and I had gone to the hottest night club in town one night. I had excused myself at one point to go to the bathroom. As I came out of the stall, I noticed this gorgeous girl, and knew that I had seen her before. I must have seen her in other clubs around town. She seemed really upset about something, and I asked if she was ok? Bonnie proceeded to tell me a story about her life, and truly concerned, I had inched closer, and our faces we not far from one another. Before I knew what had just happened, Bonnie leaned in and kissed me. I froze for a moment in time, not fully able to process what had just happened. Then I quickly pulled away. Sure, I had gotten hit on by a lot a women in the past, but none were quite as forward as this person. Bonnie was absolutely gorgeous too, which confused me even more. She was tall and her black, sassy haircut was short, and she looked to be of Latin decent. Not knowing what to do, I quickly excused myself, and headed back out to see Cory. I told him what had just happened, and of course, it turned him on immensely. He, of course, thought that I ought to go right back to her, and invite her home with us. Well, I was way too shy, and had not time to process this at all.

It seemed as though everywhere we went after that, Bonnie would be there. Although it is hazy to me now, I do know that she came home with Cory and I once. I have absolutely no recollection other than that. I am not even sure where it was that we ended up, I must have been wasted that night.

Anyways, I just needed to introduce you to Bonnie so that I can weave it into my story. Let's go back to the time period prior to moving in with Ralph. I had been spending all the time that Kaytlin was at her dad's or grandmother's place, at Ralph's house. I was still in the suite which KK and I loved. Ralph and I had had a viscous fight and I had gone home a day or two prior and did not really want to see him for a few days, while I cooled down. His ex and her sister had come over unannounced to his house a couple of evenings prior to that, and I had come into the kitchen and caught the ex on Ralph's lap. Having seen enough, I jumped in my car and zoomed off. I think I ended up at the night club, the next night. And there she was. Well, obviously, we knew each other better now, and so she stuck to me like glue that evening. As I was about to leave for the night, she told me that she had forgotten her house key, and that her mom would be sleeping now, and that she did not want to wake her up. Well, I have always had an "open couch" policy in my house, and turned no one away. I was not altogether comfortable, since I could tell she really liked me, and I am about as straight as they get.

Anyways, I did invite to her spend the night at my place on the couch, and brought her home with me. We were both really drunk, well, I was really drunk, and definitely was not feeling any pain. I recall sitting on the sectional, as she sat herself before me. She sat wedged in between the coffee table and myself, on the floor. I was more than aware that she wanted to fool around. She asked me if she could kiss me, and I told her that I was really uncomfortable about it, and that I only like men. She told me not to worry about it, and she told me that if I just lay back, relax, and close my eyes, she would make sure that nothing she did would make me uncomfortable. It took an awful lot of coaxing, even though I was plastered, but once she convinced me that she wanted me to do nothing to her in return, I finally succumbed. That night was one of the most incredible experiences of my life, because it was just so tender and so gentle and so different. Actually, there is no other way to put it...it was fantastic, so great that I actually bought her back to my room, where we lay in each others arms for the duration of the night.

Until we were rudely awakened, too early in the morning, by a loud knock on the door, which we tried to ignore, but would not go away. I threw on my housecoat, closed my bedroom door, and went to open the front door. Shit...there he stood. I had totally forgotten that he was going to court that morning, and that it was just down the road from my place. Although, Ralph had never come over unannounced before, there he was. Not being sure how to handle this or how to get rid of him, I let him in. I was still pissed off about his ex having been over. I nervously walked down the hallway in front of him, and as we came into the living room, it dawned on me. He stopped dead and stood gaping with a puzzled expression on his face. Quietly, he asked me who's the man's jacket was that lay strewn over the couch. It did actually look like a guy's coat. I cannot recall what it was I said, but the next thing I knew, he was stomping towards my closed bedroom door. Both parties definitely registered surprise as they looked at each other. No one knew what to say, so I pushed him back out, and saying "sorry" to Bonnie, I closed the door and told her to sleep it off.

Ralph and I went back out into the living room, where he told me how relieved he was that it was not another man in my bed, and how excited he was that I had a hot chick in there. The next thing you know, we were plotting to have her stay there with us for as long as we could convince her to. We both went back to the bedroom, and invited her to stay for the day and have a special dinner with us later that evening. Easy peasy...she was all for it. The next two days were a whirlwind of great food, lots of great sex, and many tangled sheets. Bonnie continued to maintain that I did not need to touch her in any way in which I was not comfortable, and took extreme delight in pleasing me. She was so into it and so good at it, that it was not long before Ralph actually became jealous. I will never, ever, (nor do I want to forget) looking down at them both between my legs, shoving each other out of the way. Cool, I thought, I've had guys fight over me before, but I had never had a man and a super beautiful woman fight over who was going down on me. They were literally nudging each other out of the way, and arguing over who did it better. I LOVED IT!!!

Anyways, that had all happened prior to us moving in together in that huge house in Panorama Ridge. Shortly after myself, Kaytlin, Ralph, and his pit bull, Brar, moved there, it was Kaytlin's fifth birthday. We decided that we would throw a double party, so we could "kill two birds with one stone" so to speak. We had Kaytlin's birthday party throughout the course of the day, and when the kids were all tuckered out, KK went over to a family members' house to spend the night, so we could carry on with our house warming party. It was a hoot. I was not strong enough in those days to say no, when Ralph had invited Christi (one of the two "shop girls") and her kids too. Of course, it had led to many, many fights up until the event, but I was too weak and lost the argument, as would happen way too often. I suppose that by today's standards this would have made me seem totally desperate. I suppose that I totally was. So, I made it a mental focus to avoid them the rest of the night, and have fun with my friends and my family, who took up most of the population there. There were, I guess, about sixty people.

I recall walking into the living room to see Leann sitting and chatting with my mom. "Well, this ought to be entertainment at it's finest," I thought, as I meandered over. In between mom and Leann sat my dad. Leann, as always, was passing the joint. My dad did not notice that I had entered the pod, when she looked poignantly at me, and handed it to him. He took a couple of hauls, and then his eyes drew up to mine, his own getting as big as saucers. "Oh," he sputtered, "is this what I think it is? I must have grabbed it absentmindedly. I don't want this," he said, and shoved it back in the Leann's direction. "How funny, how bizarre," were my thoughts, as I sauntered off.

Leann had been setting my mother straight on some matter to do with my childhood, and I wasn't into that either. I remember my brother and his new girlfriend leaned against the kitchen counter, and an all night lip lock, completely unapproachable, they were so in tune with one another. I knew this embarrassed my parents, oh so much, but then we were always good at embarrassing them.

Shit, made the mistake and looked into the kitchen, and there in the corner, were the two of them, deep in conversation, then reeling back and laughing oh so raucously with his friends, whom I barely knew, but SHE did. The slut had also sent her own kids home. "Ignore it," I thought, "there is nothing going on." "Who in their right mind would make it that obvious?" I thought to myself. I know now, that if someone needs to ask themselves all of these sorts of questions, and chooses to overlook their own gut feelings, then there is something definitely wrong! Oh...live and learn, Petra. Live and learn. The rest of the night did go without any hitches, and the Idiot did begin to migrate and stay by my side after a while. She and the rest of his friends left, and mine stayed on. We had a blast!

Speaking of hindsight, I have to interject here, that I do not regret anything I have ever done or said, in that it has made me who I am right now. Yes, I have been a mean person at times, when I haven't been outgoing and the life of the room. At times, I was also temperamental, and an outright hormonal freak, who was sometimes out of control. I think most women are, and those that are absolutely not, ever, I believe in my humble opinion may have stifled the urge their entire lives. I still have the work ahead of me to lose my anger, and get back to love. I have been through so much up until now, that there will be a second book, it just won't all fit into one. I really had only myself to be angry at, for being so weak in those days.

And so, life in Panorama with Ralph began. As I had mentioned, he was now unemployed, and ended up "on the system." Not only was I trying to break into the real estate business, in a recession, which is pretty much impossible without money, and supporting my daughter, but now I found myself supporting, not only a grown man, but a grown man with a heavy drinking problem. Ralph in turn, turned the basement of our home into a marijuana grow show. At first, I did not pay much attention, but then I realized that this was the real deal, right down to fake walls and rooms with television sets, in case anyone were ever to look through any of the windows at the front of the house. It was a very elite, professionally built (by three young men), hydroponic system. After the initial setup, I really wasn't "allowed" to go downstairs. Kaytlin, being so young, had no idea what was going on, or why she could never go downstairs. He made sure that he only went down there when she wasn't paying attention at all.

One story I will never forget, is the time that Ralph and I went downtown to go out with some friends. We ended up staying at my friend Mandy's house overnight, because we didn't want to drink and drive. We both had an incredibly strong impulse, however, to get going first thing in the morning. He was concerned about his plants, as he was only one week away from taking down a $70,000 crop. When we arrived home, Ralph immediately went downstairs to check on his plants, and the next thing I knew, he was calling me down (which never happened). When I got down there, he was crying like a baby, gaping at all the dead plants. The pump that gave the little guys water to survive had blown, and the lights, (which were now very near the plants), had burned the shit out of them. All he was able to save in the end was about two or three pounds, and there went $70,000 all in one fell swoop. Whatever proceeds he did end up with, were invisible to me, because the Idiot did not share a red cent of it. Not then, and certainly not later.

Ralph and I had quite a torrid relationship for the next couple of years. We were together for three and a half years in total. I thought that I was truly in love with this man, but in retrospect, I know now that I was in lust with him. One really huge bonus was that Ralph and Kaytlin had a really great relationship, and he really loved her, or so it seemed at the time. I am not sure that Ralph knows how to love. They were so close in fact, that I have to admit, it sometimes made me jealous. Other than her father, this was the only other male influence that Kaytlin has ever really had.

But between us, it was always up and down, and so I would sometimes escape, and sneak off to get high with other people. By that, I mean that once in a while, I would go out and smoke crack. Ralph always knew when I was high though, and I could not fool him, although I tried. See, he did cocaine, and even smoked it once in a while himself, but I seemed to care for it much more. He used it to pick up women. Most of our fights, some of them pretty intense were usually about Christi and her friend. I did not want him going over there and he of course, paid no heed.

I recall one day in particular of which I am not proud, because Kaytlin was there, and should not have been witness to this. We had had a huge volatile fight which began in the kitchen, where he made me so mad, that I threw a coffee pot across the room, aiming (but a controlled aim, if you know what I mean) at his head. I think that Kaytlin may have seen this, and she disappeared to the bathroom. The next thing I know, he had provoked me even further, and I lunged at him. The Idiot ran, and the next thing we knew, I was chasing him around and around the dining room table. I was so pissed off that had I caught him, I believe that I may well have done some damage. The chicken shit that he was however, finally escaped and hid in the bathroom with my daughter, knowing that I would not follow him in there.

Ralph was one of those idiots that declared he never hit women. I suppose that when he slammed my head into the ground, and grabbed me by the back of the hair, pulling me back up, and then slamming me into the nearest wall, and kicking me a couple of times while I was down, didn't count. I mean, technicalities that these men convince themselves of, are dumbfounding to me. That particular incident happened one night when his brother and I went out for a couple of drinks. When we got back to the house, Ralph flipped out. He beat the shit out of me (although of course, "he didn't hit me"), and when Sammy tried to help me, he turned on his own brother and beat him to a pulp. In fact, he broke some vessels around Sam's eye, and almost cost him irreparable damage. It was pretty bad.

Anyway, I will cut this long story short, because I do not think it requires much more credence. I got a call one day from Ralph's best friend, inviting me for lunch. They had been out partying together the week before, and Ralph and I had had a big fight, because he had not come home all night. Dan ended up telling me the truth that day...that Ralph had been with someone that night, and other nights, and that Christi and Ralph were positively sleeping together. Well...even when a woman knows these things deep down inside, we do not want to believe them, and so we choose otherwise. But, when his best friend puts it right on your plate, so to speak, then it is time to confront the issue once and for all.

Other than the great sex we always had, I think what I loved most about my relationship with Ralph in those days, was that he always had something to do, and somewhere to go. You know, when you sit around bored, and don't really know what to do, he always came up with something. We did a lot with Kaytlin...went four by four trucking, took her to play places, and camping and boating...it was always so much damn fun, to hang out together. Therefore...it was very hard to let go.

Again, he was just near the end of a big $$$ crop down there in the dungeon, in the house I mainly paid the rent and the bills for. I was not thinking about that though, when I made the final decision to get the hell out of there. But of course, not without some more of the volatility that follows such a break up. I was still totally in love with him, but could not find it in myself to stay, knowing beyond a shadow of a doubt that he could not keep his pecker in his pants for two fuckin' minutes. So, KK and I went to my girlfriend Carmen's to stay until we found our own place. I still, to this day, do not know why I did not force him out of the house instead, what a dumb ass. Maybe it was because I knew it would be futile to even suggest, and easier to move?

I do not know why to this day, but all in all it ended up taking me three more years to get over this guy, who had treated me so badly. During those dark days, I had to admit to myself that I was in love with him, but he certainly was not in love with me. It became embarrassingly obvious over the passing years.

The next place that I ended up at...oh wait...gotta tell you one more story, because it was a crazy day. Ralph had a really nice corvette, which he had paid thousands of dollars to get repainted. That was when he was still at his own place prior to us moving in together. It was pretty hilarious actually, because the day he went to pick it up from the shop...he went there drunk, as always, since he was rarely sober. On the way back (it had snowed a centimetre or two overnight), he hit a bloody pole about two blocks from home. Back into the shop it went...two more thousand dollars, I think to fix again. Well, this car was the Idiot's "everything." He loved that car and would not ever let anyone touch it, especially me, for I was a very heavy leaded driver in my youth.

Ha, ha. Ralph got a call one day to go to work right away. Nearing the end of our relationship, his mom had paid for him to go to driving school. My car was in the shop I think, I cannot recall for sure. The only car we had available to take him was the Vett, and since he was trucking, and going out of town, he didn't want to leave it in the lot. So...poor little Petra had to take it back home for him. "Make sure that you take it straight home, no detours, and park it," he demanded. Boy, oh boy...was that a good weekend. I didn't go home. It was out of character for me, to do something so deceitful, that I knew he'd kill me for. Nope, I took the corvette and went straight to the bar! There I ran into a friend of ours, who told me that he had to take care of some business, and had a few stops to make. Thinking nothing of it, and dying to drive the Corvette around on this beautiful sunny day...I enthusiastically agreed to be his driver. Off we headed in the Vett towards some neighbouring locals.

Well...silly, naive me, didn't really clue in until we were at bar number three, I was having so much fun. But, that was when I noticed a movement in the rear view mirror, and witnessed an angry China-man, chasing my esteemed colleague down the ally way where I sat waiting. That was when I realized that I was the fucking get a way driver. After I had made it far away from the bar, I pulled over, and demanded to know what the hell he had gotten us into? It was then that he handed me my half of the profits, and that helped a little bit, I guess. He had been running a bar pull-tab scam, for Gosh sakes. They had printed up the $500 prize tickets and were cashing them in everywhere. It looked real to me too. But, I advised, that would have to be the last bar for the day, except of course the one we were going to spend some of that hard earned money in!

The next day, I awoke feeling a bit groggy, but cheered right up when I looked out the window and realized it was another beautiful summer sunny day in the neighbourhood. Over the course of the LONG weekend, I took several road trips. I drove up to Whistler, and then to Tsawwassen. I drove to beaches, and to the mountains. I took long languishing, scenic, gorgeous, life loving drives. Those ones when all of a sudden, you feel this warmth come over you, and you have an unexplainable gratitude to be here. To be alive. So much love overwhelms you, in those moments in time, that it brings tears to your eyes. What a weekend to be alive. I did not actually ever tell the Idiot about taking his car out, until about three or four years ago.

My life after I moved out of there went totally crazy. It drove me into a downward spiral like none other. What you are about to hear next is mind boggling even to myself. How one girl could have so many things go wrong, and endure so much pain is incredulous to me. I lost control of everything. I do not in this moment even know where to begin. Allow me for a moment to collect my thoughts. It hurts as I write this book to "go there." I have come to another realization that I have told my stories over and over to my friends, and acquaintances, and even to strangers, but I was told recently that my writing, brings it to life. Make sense? So then, let's begin this part of my journey where it perhaps begins? Haha

# Chapter 6 – Life After the Idiot

My next place was what Kaytlin and I still call "the pink house." It was a basement suite right beside the railroad tracks on a somewhat busy road. Not just that, but the train ran about 50 yards from our heads in bed. The suite was new and really nice actually. I began to party more, and drop Kaytlin off to her family more. Gray and I were not those kind of people who ever used their child as a pawn, and we had become best, best, friends. Since we had split up we always still did things together with both of the kids, as much as possible. To see Braydon was a bit more difficult, because he still resided on the Island. But, Gray always shared him with me too, and we maintain a close relationship to this day. Braydon is like my own son to me.

Anyways, the pink house became quite the...not necessarily party house, but the place I resided when I really began to let loose. Kaytlin was seven years old by now. Real Estate had definitely hit the big dark hole, and I had exhausted all my funds. It became increasingly difficult to pay my rent and bills, not to mention my now growing cocaine habit. I began to get addicted, although I had always been able to "dabble" in the past. What really got my goat was when I heard that the Idiot had taken down the last crop of weed, and I did not get a single red cent from that either. Is that a selfish human being or what? Not to mention that I had to start all over because Ralph had also kept most of my belongings. But, enough of that, it is all water under the bridge now.

I sure can't say that those days were not also fun, though, because isn't that what I was trying to achieve here? There are simply too many stories to tell, and this book would be too long. The pink house is where I was at when I met this guy named Ethan. I had gone back to work at Revenue Canada for a season, and a friend I worked with there had asked me to go to this BBQ with her. I really did not feel like going at all, but felt an obligation, because she had invited me out so many times before. No sooner had we arrived, and were greeted by the home owner, than my eyes were drawn over to my right, as though by some magnetic force. There stood a guy with his back to me, and his hands casually tucked into his jeans pockets, under a great looking, white, long, cable knit sweater. Although I had not seen his face, I knew. I just knew. It was like the time that I had met Gray...love at first sight. I told the two girls walking beside me. I said, "See that guy over there, in the sweater, he is totally my type."

Well, I was really shy sometimes, and it wasn't until I had had a few drinks in me, that I was even able to look at him. I had seen his face of course, by now, and he was gorgeous, and Italian. I have always been partial to Italian men. Perhaps because that is my favourite place on Earth. I have never had a draw to go back to my native country, but I do know that I have to go to Italy before I die. That is a fact. I have many relatives left in Germany I could stay with, but have never had a desire to go. Isn't that weird? Seriously, all my childhood memories for many years were of Italy only. Memories of Germany came back to me in dreams and nightmares. Horrible nightmares. I am still not sure why that is? Maybe it was those creepy castles my parents had taken me to. I will never forget this one castle, where you entered the lobby and on one of the counters there was a glass encasement, with a little black hand in it. My mom and dad told me then that it was the hand of a little boy who had hit his mother, and his hand had fallen off. Traumatized me... you have no idea!

Another one my mom used to tell me was that if I lied, which is all I ever did as a kid, (because I feared my parents so much) if I lied, then she would be able to tell because my legs would grow shorter. One day after a long walk she caught me checking them in the mirror. Then there was the bubble gum story..."If you swallow your gum, you will end up with a gum tree growing in your stomach, that will make you really sick. The best one however, was the one where she told me that if I was a bad girl, then she would send me away to where all the bad girls go...to a place called Bella Bella. Boy was I creeped out when years later, I found out that there really is a place called Bella Bella, in British Columbia.

But enough about all that, we were discussing the day I met Ethan. We ended up together at that BBQ, and were together a lot after that. I really loved this guy, but alas, I was not ready, for I had not gotten over Ralph, not even close it turned out. Ethan spent a lot of time with me in the "pink house." It seemed to me that every time he came over, though, I could not get rid of him, and I needed time to heal. I know now that he was himself on the rebound, and had fallen head over heels in love with me, but it all happened too fast. Poor guy, he had been at my place for at least a solid week, and I had had enough. I made a big thanksgiving dinner and had my dad over (mom was in Germany), and a couple of girlfriends. I still feel bad to this day, that it was after the great dinner that I kicked him out. Well, at least I fed him first. I didn't see Ethan for a while after that, but found myself missing him. The timing was just too messy, I suppose.

Here I pause, because it is unclear to me now, where we ended up after the pink house. I know that my financial situation had gotten so bad that we had to move. I believe (see how hazy life can get when you are on drugs?) Oh, my Goodness, that reminds of THE story I forgot to tell you about Ralph and I. This was the defining moment, that one moment in time, when your whole world changes. Shit, it was before the pink house. That wasn't the first house after the Idiot at all. We had actually ended up in another basement suite prior to the pink house, and prior to meeting Ethan. There, I had started to go downhill. Now I remember how things gradually had gotten so bad. Shoot, sorry, I hope this doesn't confuse you guys too much. I often sit here in tears so big I can hardly see the keyboard as I frantically type.

At this time, Ralph and I had been seeing each other again, or was it still? I suppose we never really stopped. I was addicted to him, to the sex. It was even more exciting after I moved out. I guess he was trying even harder to impress me or something. It was while I was in this grey suite, that I had called in sick to work one bright sunny day in order to go across the line (Canada/USA border) with him in his work truck. Oh, yes, just the same as my first boyfriend (who did not work a day while I was with him), Ralph got a job as soon as I left him. Go figure. By then, I had broken up with him again, after finding out that he had been seeing one of the strippers at the bar. My whole life, I have made it a point to never date a married man, or one that had a girlfriend. I have made two exceptions. One was when I dated my realtor friend Cory, who was in a marriage of convenience, (and I truly believed that to be true) and when Ralph was with Martha (the girlfriend after me.).

So, off we drove with a big load of scrap metal, and a huge trailer on the back, hauling the same. We were headed to the USA border, and he was on a dead line. I was super excited because I had packed what I called my "slut bag." We were intending to stay in the States overnight, and head back later. Anyways, because he was trying to get to the border on time, he was going way too fast when we hit the turnpike onto the freeway. I knew it wasn't good when I felt the trailer behind us, begin to lift the truck off it's wheels on my side. Ralph had just enough time to say "We're going over," and then it all went weird. That moment in time, when everything is in slow motion, but at the same time, it all happens within the blink of an eye. The next thing I remember is seeing him laying beneath me. At first I honestly did not know if I myself was dead or alive, but then I felt my body. I screamed as I looked down and thought him to be dead or really badly hurt. "I'm ok, I'm ok," I remember him saying, and by then there were voices outside. I looked up to see my passenger side window far above my head.

Next, I saw a couple of heads peeking in, and asking us questions. They helped me climb out of the same side window since that was the only way out. I recall the heat of the stack on the semi, which almost burned me. Someone took me to the side of the road, where I shook like a leaf in the hot, hot summer sun. I couldn't figure out why I was so cold? I think behind me they were helping Ralph out of the truck, but I was unable to move, frozen in time and space. I recall a voice saying, "You are in shock, it's ok, you are alright, and your boyfriend is alright." I still wish I knew who the kind soul was, that was there for me that day. I cannot even tell you for sure if it was a man or a woman. Whoever you are, if ever you read this book, I thank you for your kindness and concern. It meant a lot. From what seemed like a great distance, I heard the sirens, knowing they were on their way to help us.

And, so, the Idiot and I were both at the hospital when the media showed up. Apparently we had made quite a mess of things, and people had been rushing to the poles to vote, at the time. Luckily, although the entire on and off ramp had to be closed until about 2am to clean up the mess (for which they had to call in large cranes and other equipment) no cars on the other side of the road had been hit and no one else had been injured. Ralph and I got released from the hospital a few hours later. I think that I had parked my car at the bar, because that is where we ended up. Oh, wait, maybe we somehow got to my house and picked up my car, yes, I think that is what happened. I think we picked up my car, and he drove (he never let me drive) to the bar, and we ended up in the lounge. I felt like a walking zombie, as I walked in, I totally remember that odd feeling that consumed me. I recall sitting up at the bar, but everything seemed to be in this strange sort of a fog. I suppose looking back upon it, that I was totally in shock.

I remember him asking me not to tell anyone what had happened, because he didn't want Martha to know that I had been with him. At the time, I could give a shit, that was the least of my worries. I was just happy to be alive. I then recall, leaving the lounge in the same zombie-like state, and he drove to the work yard close by where he had picked up the semi. The man that he really was, then actually handed me my car keys, and expected me to get myself home, as though nothing had happened. I recall feeling so completely used and abused, and so very, very little in that moment. I had no strength left to fight or even to tell him what a loser I thought he was, to do this to me.

A couple of days later, my phone began to ring off the hook. The first call I received was from a good friend of mine, who stated that I was on the television show called "To Serve and Protect." "Ya, right," I laughed and hung up. After the third call though, I had no other recourse but to believe them. I guess the media had been there while the Idiot and I were in the hospital. How it ended up on "To Serve and Protect," I am not clear, because I had thought that they only have footage of criminal cases. I suppose that maybe the wreckage was so dramatic that it made for good television. They still air it sometimes, and I still get the odd call, but I have never seen it. It was always over by the time I picked up the remote, and tuned in to the right channel.

In the meantime, though, being the person that I pride myself to be, I had phoned Martha and told her that I had been in the truck with him. I was grateful to have called her before everyone, including herself, saw it on television. Although, she was livid, she did thank me for having the guts to tell her the truth. I recall telling her one day, (for we ran into each other at the bar from time to time) that I did not feel bad for continuing my relationship with the Idiot, since she had done the same to me. I also told her that she was a fool if she thought that just because he had switched girlfriends, that he was going to keep his pecker in his pants. I suppose though, that seeing it on TV must have kept bringing it back to the surface for her and Ralph. I often got phone calls from her at four or five o'clock in the morning, threatening to kill me.

# Chapter 7 - What May Well Be "The End"

It was after the trauma of that event and the end of my contract at Revenue Canada, now cut short, that led me on a brand new path of destruction. My life was turned upside down. I had sustained neck and back injuries, a lot of muscle and tissue damage that plague me to this day. It also led me back to opiate prescription drugs, which I had not done in years. The hoops the system makes you jump through are endless, and I found myself having so many appointments with governmental agencies, and doctors, and physiotherapists, that it became a full time job. I should have gotten myself a lawyer, but I didn't. After dealing with five different government agencies to survive, I ended up a couple of years later with a whopping $10,000 payout. It wasn't even a single payout, just chump change here and there. And of course, all this aided me in was getting more deeply involved with crack and cocaine use, and partying.

I ended up hanging out with a couple of realtors I worked with who were into the crack, and needed a crack companion. I also hung out with a friend from one of the bars Ralph used to take me to, the roughest one in Surrey actually. Ross, this guy we'd met there was seriously in love with me, and was an ongoing presence in my life after the Idiot and I split up. I didn't like Ross that way though, not at all, but he always had crack. Crack, crack, crack. As soon as KK was in bed, or especially when she was away...it became the agenda. A very important agenda. I suppose because the other realtors were doing it also, (and the general public seems to hold them in such high esteem) that it made it even more okay to do, in my stupid mind.

I ended up moving out of that suite when the septic system backed up. The septic was in the back yard, which lay above my in ground suite. It was the most disgusting thing that I have ever had to endure, for it was also left up to me to clean it up. Shit came up through an outlet under my living room carpet, and up through the drain in the bathtub, and another drain in the water heater closet.

It all grossed me out so much, that we gave notice. That's when we moved to the pink house.

Alright, now that we are back at the pink house let me go on... it was a fun kooky time...I partied every chance I got, and now that Ethan was gone, and I had lost out twice, I suppose I needed to self medicate. Having been in the semi accident...the fantastic doctors put me on both Tylenol 3's and amitriptyline, which is a anti depressant given for chronic pain. There my life of real pain began all over again. I had started out with severe scoliosis, which is a curving of the spine. Mine goes in the shape of an "S." Given these issues, the tear and damage to my muscle tissue was accelerated. I have to say though, that I never did abuse these drugs, which having been a junkie is unheard of. I did not do more than a couple T3's a day. I have always been the most "in control" addict I have ever known.

I did not particularly like the landlords at this residence, and was not comfortable in this house. The funds had run out. I recall being so broke at one point that some of my friends got together and anonymously dropped off a food hamper at my door. I do not know for sure who it was, but I have my guess. I think that I am actually the richest person in that I have very good friends of twenty to thirty years standing, and in some way they have all been there for me when I needed them the most. What I think I have given them in return in loyalty and understanding, and often a lot of good advise.

The thing of it was that I was able to give a lot of solid good advice, but I myself needed saving. My closest friends did not know at the time how bad things really got for me. I feel so very, very sorry for my daughter now in hindsight. For the next few years, I was not the best mother that I could be. I see now that Kaytlin suffered in that I did not give her the attention that she needed. I became volatile and moody over time, which needs to be spoken about now, before I begin the next saga of my story. I just need to get it all out now. Kaytlin, I know that someday you will read this, and I hope that you can forgive me, because "I love you to infinity and beyond."

With the cocaine use, I became very moody, and the day after I used, I was basically useless. Kaytlin had to fend for herself way too much. I began sleeping in more, and it came to a point that I did not get up before 11am. Then there was the fact that as soon as things got too bad again, I would move, always hoping for a better tomorrow. I was running, and things progressively began to spiral out of control. I became very strict about KK's bedtime, because that would be when I could "make the call." I always "used" the second she was out the door. Kaytlin had to get herself to school at lot of the time, and often had to make her own lunches. It hurts me so much to have to tell the world how shitty of a mom I became, that I sit here now sobbing uncontollably. One thing I never did do though, was to get high in front of her. There were two slips, where I had forgotten myself, and they will be brought up later. But first, let me go on...this is where it gets difficult for me. It became the deepest darkest part of my existence thus far.

So...out of the pink house and into a old, old run down house on a busy road in the throes of Surrey. The house I rented next was my own, and not a suite, which felt good. I had a few good backyard parties there, and it was not a bad place. There was a big empty bedroom in the house, and when my little brother took ill for a while, he and his girlfriend moved in. That helped me with the rent and it was nice to have the company. I thought it would make it really hard for me to do any crack while they were around, but as you may know, there is always a way, and I had become addicted.

As before, whenever Kaytlin was away for the weekend, I would be on the phone to the dealer right away. There, in that house...it became almost nightly that I would call and have it delivered, just as soon as KK went to bed. My brother had a camper van in the driveway, and so they weren't always in the house, since they slept out there most nights. They seemed to prefer it in the van. Other than that, they turned a blind eye whenever the dealers came and went, pretending that they did not know what was going on. After the dealer would leave, I would disappear into my bedroom, and hide in there for the night. They didn't mind, because then they had the living room to themselves. And so it went for a few months.

It was in this house that I had my first overdose experience. I had been up for two days doing the stuff, as KK was gone with her dad to the Island, where he had moved, having gotten married by now. I had been invited to his wedding, since he and I would always remain best friends. It sure caused a lot of weird reactions form her friends and family, but I didn't care, and was most amused by it all. Anyways, I'd been up for two days, and had caught myself falling asleep a couple of times, with more crack to wake up to, which usually never happens. I recall that darkness had fallen again, and I remember that my roommates were out in the living room. It was then that I suppose I did a hit that was by far too big, and my body was now exhausted. The next thing I knew...I fell back onto the bed, and I knew that I was going under. Something was definitely wrong, but I was too numb and stoned to figure out that I was overdosing. I fell back against the pillows, and began to slip away, allowing it to take me...and then it happened.

I am feeling the tears well up again as I write this now. I am so lucky to be sitting here right now and telling you about it. Through my tears the keys have become blurry.

My eyes opened slowly, as though someone were forcing them apart, and there she stood...at the end of my bed. The lighting in the room was very, very dim, but she was not. There, at the end of my bed, just as real as this computer in my hands is now, stood my darling daughter. There was an aura, a bright light around her, and she stood looking down at me. She wore the most beautiful white, white dress. I cannot describe to you the look on her face, although I know that it was not fear, or anger, or distress or anything like that. It was maybe one of a deep sadness and a deeper caring. As she held out her hand to me, I slowly sat up and with all the energy I could muster, I reached out. (Shit...I am bawling like crazy now.) As I found the strength to sit, and as we reached for one another, she slowly dissipated. She had been so real, so solid...I find it difficult even now to imagine it to be real, but as I sit here, I tell you that it was. It, and she were as real as anything else in my life, as real as she is today and every other day. Somehow my little angel saved my ass that night.

Things began to unravel at this house, between my brother and I. I became more and more volatile. There was one weekend, after they had moved out again, after my brother had gotten back on his feet. He had been home after a hernia operation. One of his cats had poked some holes in my much loved water bed. It became a day of chaos, and one that I will always regret, since I know I really scared Kaytlin that day. I had decided that morning after having patched the holes, to fill my bed back up. So, in went the garden hose. Well, by the time I remembered that the bed was filling up, (after having gotten sidetracked by something) there was a fucking gushing fountain in my room. The bed had become a round blue balloon, and the water was spewing straight up into the air. What a mess! The worst part was, that I knew we were going to be moving again, and there were boxes of shit all over the room. They were now wet. Out I hauled the wet/dry vac, trying to remain calm. Kaytlin may have given you another perspective, if she were to be asked. Back and forth, back and forth, to the bathroom with the small vac, I went. I was exhausted by the time I had it all sucked up.

Then I put the hose in again, and thought to myself that I would have to make sure not to forget this time. I picked up a book and began reading, staying nearby, but in the living room. If you can believe it, I got lost in the book. Unbelievable...this time I burst at the seams. I mean, I literally became unglued. I was already in a bitchy mood, because after all that work the first time around, all I could think about was getting high. Of course, I could not, because Kaytlin was home for the weekend. Okay, so, I bit the bullet and did all the excruciating work again. I was done, again, and for the third time, I put in the hose...and oops...made the same mistake and picked up the Gosh-Damned book.

Yup, a third time, a fucking third time. I could not believe my luck...I lost it all together. In that moment, in those many moments (for the tirade seemed to last forever), I was on the teetering edge of sanity versus that simple lapse straight into the depths of insane hell. It was hard, it was one of the most difficult times in my existence, to get through. I threatened to leave and never come back. Kaytlin was scared to leave my side now, as I threatened to kill myself. I wailed that I could not go on, I kicked, I screamed, I flailed...I became an insane monster. What I must have looked like to my daughter, I do not wish to imagine.

This is the hardest part of the book to write. What she must have seen through her eyes. I am sure that my face must have been as distorted as my mind, and my thinking. I am so sorry my dear, sweet Kaytlin. I am so sorry that you had to live through this with me. I am so sorry that I could not find more control. I am eternally sorry for all of the pain I have caused you. Until this very moment I have never been able to admit it, not even to myself. Kaytlin...you must read this...you are the light of my life, and I love you like no other. I can only remember one other moment when I had been that close to the edge, and that was when Dennis and I had had a huge fight, and he tried everything in his power to push me over the edge. This time though, it was nothing but my own undoing.

While we had resided at this old house, I had been applying at Costco, which was right across the street. I had finally been hired for the Christmas season. Until, of course, Jane, whom I still believed to be my friend, talked me into taking over a house in Mission, a neighbouring suburb. The fact that I needed to run again, and figuring that I would make a lot of money, and at the same time be away from the coke and the dealers, drew me in. You see, Jane, whom I had know since 1979, (the one who had three boys with Roy) had a marijuana grow house all ready to be taken over by someone. What I didn't know was that it had already been busted a couple of times, being so "green" to the industry. I really did need the money though, and therefore it didn't take too much deliberation on my part. So, off to Mission we moved. And there went my opportunity with Costco, because as they informed me, I would have to start from scratch at a new location. Next stop...Mission...it was in November of the year 1999. The year, I wish I could forget, for oh so many reasons.

Just before I moved back to Mission, I had started seeing Ethan again. I am not sure how that came about exactly, or where, we had reconnected, but we had. Ethan was a funny bird...he was the most secretive, mysterious person I had ever met. He always came to my house, or we would meet somewhere at a pub or something, and that bothered me. I had never, ever seen where he lived, and that became a huge issue. The more I probed, the less I learned. It finally got to a point where I finally told him that I would not see him anymore until I saw where he lived. More and more now, I began to believe that he must be with someone else. Why else all the secrets? A few days later, he called and said that he would take me to his place, no problem. Like it had never been an issue, he attempted to make light of it.

So, he picked me up one afternoon, and took me to a nondescript apartment, in an older building. When we entered the dingy hallway, and he showed me around, I felt nothing of him in there. He showed me one room in particular, stating that it was his roommate's, which was filled with golf paraphernalia. Again...nothing felt or looked like him. I screamed, "Bullshit!" in my mind. In the middle of the coffee table, sat a huge candy dish...and lo and behold...it was filled with little "flaps" of cocaine. We did not stay long, nor was it comfortable, not in the least. I felt as though we had broken into someone else's apartment.

You see, it turned out that Ethan did a little bit of dealing on the side. He stated that he only brought it for his friends, and that it was his roommate who was the cocaine dealer. Turns out that that part was true, but not because Ethan did not deal per say. He just wasn't wise enough to get paid for it, and was being used. So, the long and short of it was that I figured he was married, or at least living with someone. If I had known for sure, I would have cut all ties. But, we will get back to him later. I am now going to tell you more about the time in Mission.

Kaytlin absolutely hated it there, it was the first time that we had moved that she had stated this. She did not feel comfortable at the new school, nor in the neighbourhood. I have to admit, neither did I. In Mission, I found myself so all alone. It was near Christmas time. The house we moved into was absolutely huge, a two storey, three bedroom, with a full basement. The basement had all the lights, tables and paraphernalia all ready to go. All we needed were the plants. Something did not feel right though, and it was not the fact that I had never done this on my own before. All I know is that there were a couple of guys that came by a few times, whom I vaguely knew through Jane. They paid me for part of the rent, I do not recall now how much, and told me to give them the hydro bills, which I did. It turned out a few years later (when I went to hook up power) that they had never paid the bills, and had shown me false receipts.

Well, the next thing I knew, Jane's dad's van got pulled over by the cops, loaded with grow equipment, and that was when I discovered that he had been tied to this house also. He had lived there before and gotten busted. Great...made me feel so secure. Jane, of course (having told me none of this) kept reassuring me. It was only a couple of weeks later, that Jane's brother got busted in his grow house. Along with that two more houses went down, that he had rented, using their dead brother's id. Clever, until you get caught, I suppose. The thing is that none of this had been shared with me, and these "friends" seemed to think that I was going to start the show after all that? What a bunch of bone heads! I flatly refused to go any further with this deal. Shortly after that Kaytlin came home, and told me that the girl she played with down the road told her that this house had been busted several times. What I never could and still cannot figure out is why Jane, who was supposed to be my best friend, would try to set me up in such a heat bag of a house. But the worst is yet to come.

What I have not told you yet is the fact that Gray, my daughter's father had been diagnosed with cancer three and a half years prior. The diagnosis was bad. He had been up with Kaytlin in Northern BC for his youngest brother's wedding. There, his ankles became so painful and swollen, that he came back early, and went straight to the doctor's. The prognosis and all that transpired so quickly, were worse than Gray ever let on. Now, I remember this very clearly, for it was while he and I were still living together. Gray came home one day, and told me that a fellow whom he worked closely with had "gotten zapped." He was doing that "non destructive testing" if you recall. They had gauges that measured how much radiation they were exposed to at all times. Apparently his workmate and friend had come out from behind the screen too quickly, and had gotten too much exposure.

Well, the truth of the matter seems to be that it was actually Gray who had been zapped, because that is what he told his best friend and wife, as well as his own sister. After his initial diagnosis however, he seemed to block it out completely. Outright denied having said it, as a matter of fact. Anyway, the story was that the cancer had started in his adrenal gland and carried it through the main artery into the heart. Inside his heart, was a two inch diameter tumour. Huge...right? Well, we all had no idea how huge until at least three years later, when we learned that his chances of surviving that first surgery had been a whopping 2%. Grayson, being who he was, told absolutely no one, not me, not even his own mom, how minute his chances were. All I remember quite frankly, is talking to him in the room where we waited for them to roll him into surgery. We only had a moment before his mom came in. The next thing we all knew was Gray making jokes and laughing on the gurney, as they wheeled him away.

The next few years to come for Gray, were up and down. There was radiation, there was chemotherapy, there were steroids, and meds coming out of the poor guy's ying yang. It was hard, and it always made me feel so horrid when he was living on his own, and still trying to see his kids as much as possible. In hindsight, I wish I had helped him more, with housework and stuff like that, but I have always been so lazy in these areas. His own family consisted of six kids. Well there were six kids then, another seventh offspring was announced after Gray died, so he never had the chance to meet his oldest half brother. What I began to say is that he did have a lot of help and love around him. Gray met and married Carey and she helped to take care of him after that. He even worked on and off, and whenever he felt strong enough, but I saw how he struggled. I am grateful that we always remained so close, and that we were still best friends. Gray and I confided everything to one another.

And so, the next few years had become a mirage of up and downs and setbacks, and hospital visits and stays. You see, Gray's biggest fear was that if he died too soon Kaytlin, who was only five years old when he was diagnosed, would forget him, and who he was. Braydon, was ten years old when we found out that his daddy was sick. I always reminded Gray that there were so many videos and pictures of him with the kids, and that if he were to die, I vowed to never let KK, or Braydon (for that matter) forget him. Gray, thankfully had always been what I call "camera happy." He, just like my dad, always had us posing. I hated it, but now I was grateful.

I have not seen anyone fight so hard and be so brave as he was. Gray always tried to spare us from the worst. Then came the prognosis that there was a spot in his lungs, and that triggered a distant memory almost at the same time, both for his mother and myself. We both recalled suddenly that we had initially been told, (three and a half years prior) that there had been a tiny spot. With all the chaos to follow, I suppose we had all somehow blocked it out. The same way Gray had blocked out what had really happened to him. He had, throughout his own illness gone to see his friend from work, who was in and out of the hospital, before he had died a couple of years later. It had to have been hard for Gray to watch, knowing that he had it too.

My cousin had moved up to Salmon Arm, a mid northern BC community. I'm not quite sure anymore what the occasion was, but we had all been invited up there. Since the whole family on my father's side had gone, we had all brought tents. It was fun and pretty neat, that we were all together. Let me try to recall who was there. There was my cousin and his new wife, and I believe his youngest son Andy had been born by then. There was my dad and

KK, and my aunt and uncle (whom we had flown to Canada with), and my other cousin Heidi.

We had a really good evening, laughing and drinking and catching up. I was so glad to have the family unit, for it didn't happen very often. I believe that we had arrived there at about three or four o'clock in the afternoon, and it was about 8pm when I received "the call." I think it was his mom on the other end, but everything gets fuzzy now. My heart almost stopped and my eyes must have shown my pain, as she told me that Kaytlin and I needed to come back right away. Gray was back in the hospital in Victoria and the doctors had told them that he would likely not make it this time. I remembered someone taking the phone out of my hand, and my face must have been ashen.

My dad took me around the shoulders and said," Come on downstairs with me, and let's talk." At least I think that is how it happened. He and I went down alone, and for the first time in a long time, I was so grateful that he was there. It was one of those moments when I needed him, and for once he was there, and he seemed to know exactly what to do. "What do I tell her, Dad?" I wanted to know, "How do I say it?" "What do I tell her and what don't I tell her, she is still so young?" I wanted to know. KK was 8 years old by this point. All I remember is that he kept me calm, and was there to console me, and by the time we headed back upstairs, I was able to deal. Kaytlin, having felt that something was wrong had been looking for me. I told her only that we had to go back as soon as possible, and that her daddy was back in the hospital.

I usually bring my car everywhere I go, but we must have headed up with someone else, because I had no idea what to do next. Heidi was kind enough to offer to drive us back early in the morning. We would have gone right away, but we had all been drinking. It is about a six hour drive to get back to Vancouver from Salmon Arm. We didn't stay up too much longer after that, well at least I didn't, as we climbed into the tent. Halfway through the night I awoke to battering rain, and the bottoms of our sleeping bags were wet. Perfect.

So, back we raced, and all I recall is getting to Victoria near nightfall the next night...it had been quite the trip with ferries and the such. When we got to the hospital, there was such a gloom and doom, with everyone tiptoeing around. The unfortunate thing is that his wife was not secure enough to leave us alone for even a moment. The first thing Gray said to me was, "What took you so long?" What I had learned earlier was that Gray had been in a coma. The morning on which Kaytlin and I were on route, he had snapped out of it, just like a miracle. I do not know exactly how many days I stuck around, but while I was there, Gray actually managed to make it out of bed and over to his lawyers office to sign some final paperwork. He even made it over to his brother's house for dinner, before he had to go back to the hospital. I wanted Kaytlin to visit with him as much as possible, and wasn't sure if she was really aware of what was going on. I don't think so though, because he had been in and out of the hospitals so many times before.

I will never forget my last conversation with Grayson. I wished that we would have been left alone, but his wife, along with the aid of his mother prevented that from happening. So, I recall Auntie Linda, there by the window, and his mom in the room somewhere. I recall Kaytlin was over by her Auntie. Somehow I knew this would be the last time we spoke. I sat on the edge of his bed, and leaned in ever so close, so that it was our own moment, even if the room was full of people. I told him that I was glad to see that he was not in a lot of pain. I told him that I knew how hard he had been fighting, and that we would all understand if he were to let go now. I told him that it was okay to die.

I told him that I would do my very best to be the best mother to his daughter, that I could possibly be. I knew that Gray knew that I was having some drugs issues again, but he had never said anything. He knew that I would not use around Kaytlin. I also told Gray that I would always do whatever I could in my power to make sure that Kaytlin and Braydon got to see each other as much as possible. I promised him that I would find a way to put up with Braydon's mom, even if it meant swallowing my own pride to allow the unions. We both tried so hard not to cry, for Kaytlin's sake especially, but it was impossible for him. He cried. He said that he loved me and that he knew that I would always do my best. He said that he had no doubt. He told me that he believed in me.

I then sat up straight, and glanced over at Kaytlin, who had never seen her father cry, and worried that she would be okay. I got up to leave, and as I walked to the door, Gray said, (and I will never forget this) "Have a good trip." "I will," I replied, "and you have a good trip too." He knew exactly what I meant, and I saw his face contort, just before I left the room. That had been more than I could handle. I so did not want to have to say goodbye, but am eternally grateful for having been given the chance.

Linda told me later that he had cried for at least ten minutes straight after I left. I knew in my heart that he still loved me, and that I would always love him. We had a special relationship always, even though we could not live together anymore. I was about to lose my best friend. I went out into the hall and Kaytlin followed me. I explained to her that I was going to leave her here with her family on the island, but that I had to go back now. I believe that it was a Wednesday night when I got back home to Mission. Kaytlin followed me back a few days later, but I am not sure what day that was exactly. I do know that no sooner was she back on the ferry heading home, than Gray slipped back into a coma. Unbelievable, or what?

So, it was Sunday night, and KK was due to go back to school in the morning. I awoke with a start, sitting straight upright in bed. I slowly laid my head back down, and looked over at Kaytlin, who had slept with me. since she had come back from the island. She was tossing and turning, and turning and tossing, and it was then that I knew. I looked at the clock...it was 2am, Sunday night. I knew beyond a shadow of a doubt that Gray had just died. I laid awake for the rest of the night. Morning came, and I sent Kaytlin off to school, as usual. She had only been out of the door about five minutes, before the phone rang. Again, with a sinking feeling...I knew. I slowly walked over to it, and picked up the receiver. The voice on the other end was Linda's, Gray's sister in law. She went on to tell me that he had died at about 2 am that morning. I cannot for the life of me really recall the short conversation. She asked if I could let his friends know. I went back to the couch in the living room, and sat down heavily. The rest of the morning was spent in a state of shock. The couch directly faced my huge living room window, and as my eyes drew upward and out, it dawned on me that it was a fitting day. It was one of those most incredibly dark, gloomy, rainy days, where the rain literally came down in sheets. The sky was so black that it was almost dark outside.

And there I sat looking out, in a stupor. I have no idea how long I sat there like that. The only thing that kept reeling through my head was the thought, "How am I going to tell Kaytlin?" "How the hell am I going to tell this poor innocent eight year old girl that her Daddy has just died?" "What the heck are you going to say?" I thought, "and how are you going to say it?" "I will have to try my damnedest not to cry," I thought. It just kept playing over and over again, swirling in circles in my head. "How am I going to tell my daughter that her Daddy is dead?"

It plagued me...it drove me nuts, I did not know what to do. I did not know how to act. I could not let go of the thought. I just simply couldn't quit agonizing. I did not want to be the one to have to do this. "This is a moment in time that she will never, ever forget," I thought. "She will carry this for the rest of her life, and I had better figure out exactly what I was going to say to her, and exactly how I was going to tell her." ...and all of a sudden, just as I looked up through my tears, (that I did not even know were streaming down my face) just as I looked upward to the sky...the darkest clouds I have ever seen, suddenly, miraculously, parted. I saw it happen, as though in a dream. The brightest ray of sunshine I had ever seen shone through, and shone directly on me, sitting on the couch in my living room. At the same time, I felt a serenity and a calm wash over me, like a warm fuzzy blanket. Then as clear as a bell, a voice inside my head...his voice...said to me, "Don't worry, you will figure out a way." And I knew beyond a shadow of a doubt that my beloved Gray was there in that room with me. He was here to hold my hand.

I think that I remained sitting on that couch for the rest of the afternoon. I do not remember ever getting up, and I was calm. I knew that I did not need to think about it anymore...that it would come naturally.

And then there was the little knock at the front door. The knock made by a little girl's knuckles, and there she was...home from school. I got up, brushed myself off, and went to answer it. The sun had come out and stayed, for I remember it shining upon her. She stood there in front of me, looking much smaller than I remembered. "Hey baby dolly," I said, "how was your day?" She looked up at me, and directly into my eyes, and said, "My Daddy died, didn't he?" I just nodded...thinking, "He was right, I didn't even have to tell her." I had worried and agonized for nothing. "Yes," I said, "your Daddy died. Auntie Linda called me after you had left for school." And with that I took her in my arms. We walked together slowly to the living room, where she sat on a stool quietly. She looked so very small and so very frail. And there she sat and cried...and cried...and cried. She cried harder than I had ever seen her cry before, and my heart absolutely broke for my little girl. If only I could take the pain away...if only.

An hour or so later, the phone rang. On the other end was a friend of Gray's that he had gone to school with. They went back as far as kindergarten together, and it was also Grant whom he had recently worked with. Grant's uncle owned one of the NDT testing companies, and Grant had gotten Gray "through the doors" initially. I was a bit surprised to hear from him, since it wasn't a usual call. He told me that he did not want me and Kaytlin to be alone today, and that we should come over. He lived nearby with his wife and two daughters. I had not really thought about it, and he convinced me to go over there, and we could spend the night. It made sense to me, and so I went with the flow.

Kaytlin and I packed up an overnight bag, and headed out. I remember, now, as I write this that Kaytlin had some trepidation, and had said she didn't want to go. His wife made a beautiful dinner, which I didn't taste. Then the girls went off to go to play somewhere, and we sat around the kitchen table and had a few drinks. Before long, time had passed, and everyone was tired, so we put the girls to bed downstairs, and then Melanie also turned in. That left Grant and I alone in the kitchen.

We sat and chatted for awhile, I having lost all sense of time. I think it was nearing 2 am, when I rose from the table to go to the washroom. I think Grant was getting another beer out of the fridge, and as I walked past him, he caught me and pulled me into the kitchen. I found myself up against a cabinet or wall or something. I don't know, and the next thing I realized, he was trying to throw me over the kitchen table, bending me backwards, into an impossible position. I thought my back would snap, as he tried to grope me. I do not know how I did it, but something inside me made me stay completely calm. Calm, as though nothing out of the ordinary were occurring here.

I looked up into his eyes and they were completely vacant. Grant was not in there, he was gone, I realized. And so, as though on autopilot, I called him by name. I saw the whole scene as though out of my own body. I called him to look into my eyes, and when I knew I had his attention if only for that split second, I said quietly, "Grant, Gray is watching you right now. He sees what you are doing." I watched calmly as he returned. As though in a trance, he let go, and it was over. I swiftly exited stage left.

I went to the bathroom, and when I came back out, I silently went to the kitchen, looked down at him, and told him to go to bed now. "If you don't, I will tell your wife what you just did," I said. I went downstairs and hid amongst the kids, and stayed "eyes wide open" until the light of day. I got Kaytlin up and dressed as quickly as possible, and making some sort of excuse, we left. What a day!

Life and finances continued to go downhill. I have to tell you guys about this one morning, a month prior to Grayson's passing. I woke up on a dark and rainy day, and I felt so lost and so lonely. Friends had not really come out to see me in Mission, since it was too far for them to drive. I had no job, everything we owned was still in boxes. I had not been comfortable here from day one, even though we were in a really nice house. Gosh, I'd even bought some speed from one of the guys that had come over to talk about the upcoming "grow show." No actually, I think I had met this guy somewhere, in a bar one night or something. Things are getting dimmer and foggier in my head now. For a few weeks running, I would do some crystal meth in my special glass pipe (always had my paraphernalia stash), and play Kaytlin's Nintendo, as soon as she left for school. That became something new, since I had only ever gotten high when she had stayed at her dad's or when she was asleep for the night. But the meth was cheap and kept you high all day.

Anyway, there was this one morning in there somewhere, about a month after Gray died, as a I was saying, and I was antsy, lonely, and depressed. I had absolutely no money, not a dime to my name, and I needed cigarettes. I had been smoking since I was sixteen years old. I really wanted a drink to kill my pain, and I certainly couldn't afford the vices I truly craved. I looked around the boxes that were piled almost to the living room ceiling, and my eyes stopped on the brand new TV Gray had given us. I tried to lift it, my intention being to take it to a pawn shop that I had seen downtown. Man, was this TV ever heavy! So heavy that I could not carry it on my own, down the front steps and through the yard to the car. My eyes scanned the room and rested on a chair with rollers. I lifted the big bulky TV onto the chair, and it was a bit tipsy due to its size. Of course, by the time I made it to the front door, it had started raining bullets. The stairs were difficult, and the whole thing became one of those hair pulling stupid ordeals, at which point you hope and pray that someone you know does not see what you are doing. I somehow got the thing to my car, took it downtown, and parked. A guy walking by helped me carry it into the store. By this time, I had no shame left, and now I wanted that damned drink even more.

Oh, by the way, before I went to all this extreme, I had phoned my "friend" Jane to come out and see me. Her response was that "she could not deal with it," (meaning Gray's death) She said no. I begged her. I told her how I was feeling, and that everyone else I knew was either at work or could not be counted on to come all the way out there to see me. "Great friend," I thought, "especially since I took her to her dead brother's grave sight every year to "give him a drink." I had always been there for her, even if it was five o'clock in the morning. I was always there for my friends, and Jane was one of the needier ones. I was always there for her, no matter what. I had seen this side of her before, but it did not hurt as much or as deeply, as when I really needed her.

Anyway, that day I got a cheap bottle of wine and some smokes and went back home and played Nintendo on the small TV. We did not have cable anyway since I could not afford it. I had never, ever been this broke and destitute in my life, and it was really hard to take. In the end I lost that television set, because the pawn ticket expired, when we were on the island for the funeral.

Okay, so things are scattered in my head right now, and I know that I'm jumping around a bit here, or rather a lot. That is because my life is now spiralling out of control, and that, my dear friends, (which you now are, if you've stuck with me this far), is exactly what it feels like. You start waking up, and sometimes not being sure what planet you are on. Ethan, whom I spoke about earlier, you know the guy form the pink house, whom I had fallen in love with at first sight. Him? Well, he'd been coming around sporadically, but there was something in between us now, a distance. We did not have the same closeness we had before. If you could call it close, for in hind sight, we never really knew anything about one another. And it wasn't me, it was him, and all the secrets. He did not know how bad my habit was by now, and I tried really hard to never ask him for a "flap," in order to maintain my own secret. We had done it together a couple of times, but he would do one or two hoots, and the next thing I know he just watched me do it, or he would leave. So, it was uncomfortable. Very uncomfortable.

Christmas was the weirdest loneliest, most fucked up Christmas of both mine and Kaytlin's life thus far. My fault. Gray had died on December 6, 1999. I always remember it because it is what the Germans call "Saint Nicklaus Tag." That is where all the little boys and girls leave their shoes on the stairwell at bedtime. By the next morning, Dec. 6, they would be filled with candy from "Saint Nicklaus." All I remember is that somehow I had picked up a tree, and it was Christmas eve, which is when we open presents and celebrate. I always leave the stocking for Christmas morning, so Kaytlin has something to open then. Somehow, I had convinced Ethan to come over and spend it with us. I recall it took some convincing on my part.

I made the usual...German potato salad and European wieners. My mom has made this every Christmas eve since I can remember, and I still carry on the tradition. One thing my mom did very well was "occasions." She always made Christmas, and Easter and birthdays, so special. She always had such a warm and loving touch in her organization of these events, and that is the only time I felt that motherly warmth. She truly enjoyed it. I recall that I had spent $60 which I could ill afford on a tiny bottle of special cologne for Ethan. I have no idea what I got KK. After dinner and present opening, and after she had gone to bed, we sat up and drank. I think he had some blow and we did some lines that night, but I'm not sure. All I know is how disappointed KK was in the morning when I had forgotten to hang the stockings. I realize in writing this book that I really failed her as a mother after Gray died. I should have been there for her more, rather than licking my own wounds, and creating this horrible spiral, but I was obviously lost and therefore swallowed up by it.

Ethan didn't stick around long, and left quite quickly in the morning. After I saw that he had left his gift on the table, I was really sad, because it had been sort of a test. I figured if he was married, how would he be able to wear it? Well, I figured, I was right. Merry fucking Christmas! I do not even remember at all now what we did on that day. Not at all.

The next thing that comes to mind after that Christmas, is New Years Eve. A friend of Carmen's was having a house party, and Ethan and I had been invited some time back. I called him, and for some reason he did not have his vehicle. I think he was trying to back out, which he did often. So, I told him that I had no problem picking him up "at his place." "This ought to be interesting," I thought. I did not give him an exit this time, I just had to know more. And so, New years Eve, I drove from Mission to Burnaby (a fair distance) to pick him up at an address he gave me. He made it a point to mention that had moved there with another friend.

When I got near, I drove slowly down the road looking for the address. Suddenly, he appeared out of nowhere, walking nonchalantly down the sidewalk, kitty corner from "his house." I slowed and let him in. "I just went to the liquor store on foot to save you the trip," he said. "Shit," I thought, "he's lying to me again!". "Well, let's go in and meet your roommate for a minute then," I said. He made up some lame excuse like he's tired or napping or something, I don't recall. Duped again, but I wasn't going to let it ruin my night. So, off to the party we went.

Now, as I've said I had known Carmen a long time. One thing she always said to me whenever we went anywhere together, was "how many people do you know? Everywhere we go people know you." And it was true, and still is. I know a lot of people. I am a social creature, and get along with people of any age, stature, and colour, equally. I just love people. So, to cut a long story short, internet dating had just arrived, and Carmen had been talking to this guy online for like six months, but she would not allow herself to meet him. So, Sharlene, the friend having the party, got a hold of him, and invited him to the party. It was just after midnight when he walked in with a guy he presented as his best friend. Before Carmen even had a chance to meet her "friend," his buddy noticed me, and exclaimed his surprise. We hadn't seen each other in some time, and again the poor girl, was dumbfounded. "Jeez, Petra, she said...who don't you know?" It was really good night, and Eli and I got along really well. It was always hard to get him out amongst others, and I was just glad to be out with him.

Shortly after New Years that year the insurance on my car ran out, and I simply had no money to re insure. I still did not have a job, although I don't recall going out and trying to get one either. Ethan had a pressure washing company, and he focused on big semi trucks and trailers. He had taken up making his own soap and caustics, because the stuff on the market was simply too expensive. He had an idea that he would pay for my insurance, and pay me a sales commission, if I used my vehicle to sell his soaps.

So, anyway, I had just picked up all the soap, had already spoken with a couple of businesses, and the back of my little blue Sprint was loaded. My friend Carmen called, and we had decided to meet at a pub up by her place in Surrey, for a weekly crab feast. I took Kaytlin with me, as she was going to see the boys and Carmen had a sitter for them all. There had been light dusting of snow on the roads, and it had turned to an icy slush. I remember that it was rush hour on a Thursday late afternoon, when I was coming upon a light. The light turned yellow, and I tried to stop, but the car, (which needed new brakes and tires) just kept going, as though I had not even hit the brakes. In front of me I watched in horror as a huge supped up pickup turned into the intersection to make a left turn in front of me. Again, I tried the brakes, to absolutely no avail. "Hold on," I screamed at Kaytlin, as we collided right into his passenger's side. We had hit hard...really hard. I looked up, and the first thing I saw was the completely shattered windshield in front of Kaytlin, and I think I began screaming. My eyes were drawn like a magnet to her face, which was completely covered by her little hands. I thought her face had met with the windshield.

The next thing I remember were three men pulling me out of the car, and another helping Kaytlin out the other side. I looked vaguely at the car, and realized that my engine was now right up to my windshield. I freaked, I screamed, I cried, and then I saw that Kaytlin was okay. I ran to her and took her in my arms, and the kind men helped us to a gas station. They called the police and ambulance I suppose. I have no idea what was going on around me. People kept handing me napkins, because some soap bottles had broken open in the car and it was all over the side of my face and neck. The ambulance came, and took Kaytlin and I to the hospital a short while later. I could not move my neck...I was so scared. I was more grateful than I have ever been, that Kaytlin was okay. All she got was a burn on her hip from the seat belt.

Now what I had not told you was that shortly before this all happened, Ethan and I had decided to call it quits, and just be friends. I was devastated, for I truly loved him, but again, I assumed it was because he was married, that he had decided to go back to her or something. What had happened was, that Ethan had called me to meet him at a pub a short while before this incident. I had been over at my girlfriend Jane's. Sorry that I am jumping around again...but it is coming back to me in fragments, and out of context. Anyways, I met him and we had a couple of drinks, when suddenly his phone rang. Something about the call, which he usually made sure not to pick up in front of me, made me suspicious.

As much to my surprise as to his own...I snatched the phone right out of his hand. I asked who it was on the other end. "Wanda," she replied, "who are you?" "Wanda, I have to tell you how very sorry I am," I said. "If I had any idea that Ethan was with somebody else, I would not be here. I did not know about you, because he refuses to tell me anything at all, and had I known I would not be seeing him, just so you know that." With that I handed him back his phone. He ended the call quickly saying he would explain later. I stood up. "Where are you going?" he asked. "Home," I responded. Out I walked, and he followed me to the parking lot. His truck was parked near my car, and he followed me, playing stupid. I said, "Okay, Ethan...here it is then...the ultimatum...or let's just call it the end...either you go home with me now (and end it with her), or you go home to her." He looked into my eyes as I sat in my car, and he knew I meant it. Without a word, he turned and walked to his truck, and painstakingly slowly he pulled out of the parking lot. Just like that...gone. "This cannot be real, I thought, he'll come back." I do not know how long I sat there until I realized that he was not coming back. "So...end of that chapter," I thought.

So, (getting back to the accident) when he had called and asked me to work for him, it was only a business deal. Now, here I laid in the hospital, in a neck brace, with my daughter looking down at me...her own father dead. The doctor was so very concerned with the skin on the side and back of my neck and face, more than the fact that I could not move my neck. I questioned it, and he brought me this huge medical journal, and read out to me why it was he was so filled with concern. You see, one of the bottles, (the one that had slapped me upside the head) had a caustic material in it. When this meets your bloodstream, there can be toxic effects to a human body. I was told that I would be released and needed a ride home, after they checked my neck and it seemed okay. Just some whiplash...lucky. I asked Kaytlin to give Ethan a call, and see if he could pick us up. Oh...the best part was when the cops showed up and give me a whopping ticket...and told me it was my fault. No questions as to what had happened...just accusation...right there by my bedside.

And so, "my dark knight in dull armour." showed up to rescue us. I will never forget the conversation in the car. It went like this: "Well, now I have lost everything. I just gave up the house, I have just lost Gray, I now have no car and therefore no job, and my boyfriend has left me. I have nothing left," I wailed. "Nothing." And out of the back seat came my little angel's voice, "Well, you still have your looks mommy, and I think you are very pretty." "So sweet...out of the mouths of babes," I thought.

The next morning I awoke in the arms of Ethan, and as I looked adoringly up at him, he gasped. "Well, there go your good looks too," he said. I jumped out of bed and ran to the mirror. The caustic soap had burned my whole neck, and the side of my face and chin. So, now I truly had nothing. Well, I had my KK, and that is really all that mattered. I had not gotten her hurt or killed her in that accident. For that I have never been more grateful.

So, there I sat, all alone, in my stupid house in Mission, and now I did not even have a car. I had no idea what to do next. I knew that I could not stay at this horrid house, and those idiots still expected to grow there. Not only had Jane not come out to see me after Grayson died, but she did not go to his funeral either. The two, of course had gotten to know each other quite well, over the years. Had I listened, I would have a criminal record today, just like she and her entire family have now. "What to do now?" I wondered. I did not even have the money to move. After Gray had died, I went to Kaytlin's school and asked that they hook her up with a counsellor. I met the counsellor myself, and she was a super nice young girl. Shitty thing is though, that this sweet girl, did not have the courage to bring up KK's dad's death, not even once. Instead she and Kaytlin would go out for ice cream. Kaytlin hated that school, and did not really connect with anyone there. She hated Mission, and obviously we had to get the hell out of there. But how, I had no money left to move.

After I had mulled it over, I somehow set it all up. My parents actually stepped up to the plate (for a change) and helped me get my stuff (most of it) out of that house. I had asked my sister and brother in law if I could bring it all to their place, and have a weekend garage sale. They said, "okay." Drake and Andrea have and always will be there for Kaytlin and I. Lauren (KK's closest cousin) is only six months older than Kaytlin, and her brother Daryl is one year younger. I had really nice furniture, but I had a lot of it, and now we were rendered homeless, and so there was nowhere to put it. I remembered that it was a sunny weekend in February when all this transpired. We got back out to Surrey on a Friday, and I had given Ralph, my ex, a call to go out for some drinks, so I could get my mind off things. Kaytlin stayed of course, at Drake and Andrea's.

Ralph came to pick me up, and then we picked up another friend of his, whom I had never met. The three of us went out, and ended up at a few establishments. Ralph was buying, of course, since I had no money, and I got absolutely hammered, when he started buying shots. It was one of my most drunk experiences ever, since I always liked to maintain my cool, and to have my wits about me. That is why I never really went overboard with the drugs, because I was not a glutton on them, like everyone else I knew. The difference between me and other drug users, is that I have self control, and know my limits. Who wants to be hammer head drunk, especially if you are a female? Well, that night I was hammered beyond belief.

I know that Ralph ended up taking me back to his place, although I asked him to take me back to Drake and Andrea's. I had the garage sale early in the morning, but he wasn't listening, and we ended up in this tiny little run down house, where he now resided. I think that the living room and bedroom were one, but that is where we stopped...on the big bed in the tiny living room. All I wanted to do was go to sleep, knowing that tomorrow would be so hard, hung over. Yuck. Ralph, however, had other plans. He would not stop groping me, even though I told him I was not interested. The next thing I knew, he was on top of me. "No," I said, "I don't want to do this, and this time I really do mean it, Ralph." You see, Ralph was one of those guys that thought that "no really means yes." Not this time, I made it clear, that this time I really did mean no. But Ralph wasn't listening, and he took me by force. He just took me, and I did not have the strength to fight him off. I have heard it called "date rape," and there is no other word for it. He raped me that night.

The next morning was beyond difficult, I was so very hung over, I did not even have the strength to barter. I let all my furnishings go for far too cheap. But I just wanted it done and over with. There was still stuff left over after that weekend, and I had to find a way to get it all out of there. That was not easy either, when you have no money, and no vehicle. Most of it went to charity, and the rest ended up in the garbage. My brother and sister in law had been more than patient, having all the junk in their yard for a couple of weeks. And with that our pitiful Mission life finally came to an end.

# Chapter 8 – Mission ends.

From there we ended up once again on Carmen Lake's doorstep. Carmen has truly always been there for us, for Kaytlin especially. She is a part of their family for sure, and will always be close to the boys, I'm sure. And so, with only the clothes on our backs, we were welcomed once again, with open arms. Thank Gosh for good friends. I have four really good friends of many years standing. They have always been there for me, and they never judged me. Well, that's not true, one of them is more judgemental than my own parents, but she can't help herself, she was raised by German parents also. I have always been there for my friends, whenever they needed someone to talk to, or needed a shoulder to cry on, I was there.

I enrolled Kaytlin in the school that Carter and Jake went to, and she loved it there because she already knew so many kids. You see, unlike myself, Carmen, the Mother of all mothers, stayed put in the same neighbourhood. Heck, she still lives in the same hood! It was great being there with all the warmth that was shown to us, but it really was a small place. I slept in the living room, and Kaytlin slept in the bottom bunk in the boys room. Jake, whose bunk it was, slept with his mom, which had been the case anyways. Jake was just a little tike then...he was in a walker, I remember very well. I was standing in the middle of the living room, one sunny day, and Jake was on the other side of the room in his walker. The next thing I knew, I watched in horror, as a goldfish jumped out of a hanging fish tank, that my brother had made for Carmen. The little fish landed right on Jake's walker table. It seemed that time had frozen, as I watched in horror as he picked it up in his pudgy little fist, and shoved it into his mouth. Jake had eaten the kid's pet fish!

For me, it was horrible staying there, because how the hell was I going to use? I really wanted to get high and had to find a way, no matter what. I had gone job hunting right after we moved in, and had acquired a position for the tax season at a local accounting firm. It did not pay well, but it would have to do, and I had to start saving quickly for our new place. Carmen did not let me pay her anything for rent, and I just pitched in on the food bill. But, how the heck was I going to manage getting high? And so...once a week or so, I took a big risk, and there were some uncomfortable moments when she must have known what was going on. You see, Carmen worked at the hospital. She would get up at 3:30 am and go to work, come home at 1 pm, have a nap, make dinner, and go to bed by 9 pm. Pretty much clockwork, this sweet woman was, and still is. Carmen has been on the same schedule as long as I can recall.

Man, was this one ever tricky, even for an addict! I could not have someone coming over after she had gone to bed, because that would wake her up (just believe me here), and so I would have to call my dealer to arrive earlier, when she was distracted with the kids, or in the shower. I had to try to convince the guys I dealt with that timing was important. Then, I would listen, attentively for him to pull up, and find an excuse, if anyone paid attention, to go out to the garage, where the exchange was made. She caught us a couple times, and I made up some story.

Now, the harder part came. I had to wait for the whole household to go to bed, then take the giant risk of cooking down the crack on the stove, always putting a kettle or something in front of the spoon, in case anyone came out of their rooms. Strange thing is that no one ever did, not once, that I can recall. After I had cooked it and gotten into my little black container, I would sneak off to the bathroom. I would try to be so quiet, so that they didn't hear how many times I would go in there. Sometimes I would tweak so bad that I would sit there on the edge of the tub or the closed toilet seat, and shake like a leaf, hoping and praying that they could not smell it, or hear the lighter. I would imagine...(well, it isn't really imagining when you are high on this drug, but it is so hard to explain it). It is kind of like you could see them coming through the door and then standing over me, sadly looking down. It almost seems real, but you still know it is not. But it is a fear that grips your heart so hard, that your body goes rigid, so much so, that your muscles, and teeth hurt from the clenching. Your heart beats crazily out of your chest, your breathing becomes kind of shallow. Then you realize that you are holding your breath, and then you remember that you have to breath. It is not a great feeling, and it is not the reason that you want to do the drug so badly.

What keeps you coming back is the thought of that feeling that the first hit, that first rush gives you. It is like no other, but then, sometimes, often, the first hit is a letdown, a disappointment. So you chase it, trying to get that feeling that the first hit was supposed to provide, the one that you had anticipated since this morning, for Gosh's sake. Then, sometimes you get a hit that makes you shake and quiver, and hyperventilate. It's all nuts when you look back at it. And yet, I still want it back sometimes. There are still times that I dream about getting high, but it doesn't happen as often as it used to. I don't know if it is just me, (and I have asked a few addicts, and they have the same "problem") but whenever I have dreamt of getting high, I cannot get high in my dream. I always thought that was kind of weird, and definitely a rip off. I wonder why that is, that you can't get high in your dreams?

It would have been so much easier to stay there, if only I had had a car to get away in. But, it kept my usage down to only once or twice a week. When I got the accounting job, my employer was kind enough to pick me up on the way to the office. After work, I generally had to take a bus. Oh, how I hated buses. They make no sense. Here my office was on one of the busiest streets in Surrey, but rather than be able to take a bus going towards our place, I would have to take one going in the exact opposite direction, heading away from us. Then I would have to walk over to another bus stop, and catch a second bus, and it took about one to one and a half hours to get home. Home was a five minute car ride away! The bus system in the Greater Vancouver Region still sucks butt to this day.

Our next place, once I had earned enough to pay the deposit and rent again, was not far from Carmen's so that I would not have to move KK out of her school again. I think, no I know, that the most horrible thing I have done to her is move her around so much. She never really had a chance to connect with other kids. I feel bad for that, and so many other things. I wish I had a do-over. Since I have been admitting all these terrible mothering skills now, for the first time, I have called my daughter a few times, and taken full accountability. I have apologized to her for not being there in the capacity that she needed me to be. I was so wrapped up in my own pain, that I did not see hers. Everybody has always assumed that Kaytlin has dealt with her father's death so well, but I know that she hasn't yet. For years, knowing that my job as a mother was lacking, I have asked countless friends and family to be there for Kaytlin, to become friends with her, and to help guide her. No one has ever stepped up to the plate. The only one who was ever there for her in that way, was Ralph, but as soon as we split up, their relationship ended also. I just wish he had not made her so many promises, coming out of it. I think she still waits for him to come around, and be her friend again.

The next place I rented, was a dark, dark basement suite dungeon. I hated it, but it was all we could afford, that was close to the school. When we lived there, my drug use went way up. In fact, I began doing it everyday. The fact that Carmen lived so close, and I could often send KK over there after school…allowed me to do it in the middle of the day. My accounting job had ended, since it was seasonal, and I began looking for new work. There was that time span in between though. I would get up with Kaytlin in the morning, take her to school, and on my way back home, I would call the dealer. I would then have to either "come down" before she got home, or line her up to go to Carmen's. I was getting sick…I was becoming a desperate addict at her finest. One day I got a call from a realtor I used to work with, Mack. I suppose that an addict feels out another addict, and before I knew it, he was coming over a few times a week, with the goods.

Sometimes KK would even be home, and we would sneak off to the bathroom, while she wasn't paying attention. Sure, she asked what we were doing in there. We assured her that we were just chatting and having a smoke…because we couldn't smoke in the house, and there was a window in there. Lame excuse if you think about it. I went in that bathroom a lot, because sometimes he would get a call, and leave some in there for me. I would hide it under the sink and sneak in, on and off. I hated to get high when Kaytlin was around though, because it was too hard to try to pretend to be straight. So, I told Mack that we couldn't do that anymore. He would then come over when KK wasn't home.

The rest of the time, I would anxiously wait until it was Kaytlin's bedtime. If she said she wasn't tired, I would let her read for a while before bed. She knew by now, since I had to be really strict about it, that she was not to come out of her room. Often times I could not wait any longer, and I would call the dealer even before she had gone to bed, trying to time it, so that she would see or hear nothing. I'd watch like a hawk out of the living room window, and when they pulled into the driveway, I would get to the door, which was thankfully in a short hallway behind the kitchen door. I would get to the door before they could knock, hold my fingers to my lips, so they didn't say anything, make the exchange, and quietly go back into the kitchen. Kaytlin's bedroom was right off the kitchen. Now I had to cook the stuff, hoping that she was sleeping. After a while, it got easier cooking it on a spoon in front of the fireplace where I would smoke it, and blow the smoke up the chimney. I had not unpacked the boxes, and did not intend to, for I hated this dark suite. I would use the boxes to strategically hide behind, so that if she were to get up, I would hear her before she could get to me. That happened a couple of times, and that was scary. I always had the little black box with the goods hidden behind another box, so there would be nothing to see.

Even being high, this entire procedure would make me feel so dirty and so fucked up, because I could not deny it anymore. I was a freaking mess. I had never smoked the shit while my daughter was there before, and now I was even smoking it when she was awake, for Gosh's sake. I disgusted myself, I could not look into a mirror anymore, and I was losing weight, and beginning to look like a crack head.

Then, I began to think to myself...not only do I need to get the fuck out of here, but I need to get my daughter out of the city. She was ten years old by this time, and I did not want her subjected to the drugs and gangs at the schools. That is the age when they start recruit in Surrey. The fact that we had moved around so many times, left Kaytlin very vulnerable. Basically...it was high time to run again.

And so I began planning towards moving to Australia. Remember, my friend Sharlene, who had helped me raise KK at birth? Well, she had gotten married by now, and her husband and she owned a pub and motel business. Yes, Australia, sounded nice. Sure, in drugged out lala land maybe. It turned out after some investigation, that I was not able to enrol Kaytlin in the school system there. Not without a lot of money anyways. Australia protects its job market, and does not cater to single, unemployed outsiders. Then, I thought, well, we would move back to where I was raised, in Tsawwassen or Ladner. They were much quieter suburbs, outside of Vancouver. And so, with that in mind I began to seek employment in those areas.

Guys, I don't even know when it was exactly, that I discovered that I was pregnant. How could this have happened, I was usually so careful? Had I forgotten a pill, was I even on the pill? I do not remember clearly, but I was...I was fucking pregnant. Not only was I pregnant, but I was about four months along, by the time it occurred to me! Just like with my first pregnancy, I still had my period and everything seemed otherwise normal. I wish I could remember with clarity how I found out, and what led me to it, but alas, I do not. I was astounded by the news, and began fervently making appointments to ascertain what I should do. But four months? Holy shit how could this have happened?

I had been seeing Ethan, on and off, and he was the only guy I was sleeping with. Oh, except for the night that Ralph took me by force... What the hell was I going to do now? I was lost. I called Ethan, and he was right there. Ethan helped to guide me through the steps I needed to take. I told him that I thought it was his, and he said he did not think so, because of the timing. What I realized again at that point, was that he had always known my menstrual cycles better than I. I think that over the years maybe, he had taken personal inventory, as to get no one pregnant? But only he can answer that.

So, off to the doctors, I went again, and explained that it could be one of two fathers, and that it was imperative to my decision making to know who for sure. All this took another few weeks to accomplish, and I was now almost five months into my pregnancy. Luckily, as with Kaytlin, I did not show at all, even though I weighed only about 100 lbs. I did know one thing, I would not keep it if it belonged to Ralph. I did not want him tied to me the rest of my life, and there would be too many complications, and upheavals. That much I knew. Ethan told me that if he was the father, he would stand by me, and be with me. I do not know why I actually believed that, but I did, and I hoped that it was his. Kind of...I knew that there would be great risks, if I were to go through this pregnancy, because of my drug use. All of this was driving me nuts!

Finally, I got a call from my doctor, and rushed down to his office. After I left there, (maybe he had taken me there, can't remember), I recall very distinctly sitting in a neighbourhood pub. We were sitting up on high stools at one of those high round tables. I had to tell Ethan that it was not his child, and it was not easy for me. I told him that I wanted it to be his so badly. He told me then that he had known that it could not be his. I had no idea at the time, how much it had hurt him. The fact that I had even been spending time with my ex, had hurt Ethan.

So, now the hard part. They would only do an abortion up to three months, previously. These laws had just changed (and it ended up being only a short window), and they would now do it, up to five months along. If I was to go through with an abortion, I would have to make up my mind now. And so, I did. There was no way I wanted Ralph's child, possibly to be born messed up, or addicted. I would like to believe that I would have stopped using, had it been Ethan's. I hid my drug abuse from him, but I would have told him the truth, I am quite sure.

I set up the date of "procedure" at the women's hospital downtown. I took Kaytlin over to stay with Carmen for a few days. I did not want her to know what I was about to do. No way! I made arrangements to stay at Mandy's, and she also took time off of work to take me to the hospital. I have always been so blessed to have friends that I could count on, and I sure appreciated it now. When we got to the hospital, they said that because I was so far along, (which I tried so hard not to allow myself to think about) I would have to dilate a lot, for them to get it out. They explained to me that I would have to insert (into my vagina) four of these "seaweed sticks," explaining that they would swell up enough to open the cervix. With that they set up another appointment for the next morning, and sent me home to "swell overnight."

Well, needless to say, I got no sleep whatsoever that night. I was in so much pain. It was excruciating. These seaweed sticks were throwing me into the throes of labour pains. They were no different than the pains I went through when I was about to give birth to Kaytlin. Finally, as I lay there in pain, Mandy got up. I waited for her boyfriend to leave for work, before I rose off the living room floor, where I had been "sleeping" on a mattress. Mandy looked at me and gasped. I followed her eyes, which were clearly on my belly. Oh my Gosh! I had not ever seen anything like it. Holy shit, I was bigger than I had been, moments before I gave birth to my first born. Mandy, (to this very day) still has the picture she took of me in my grey and pink raw silk shirt (see how clear that image is?) that day. I have never seen the picture, and I am not sure I will ever want to see it.

The rest of the morning seem surreal to me, even now. I recall Mandy stopping the vehicle somewhere, and getting out. I picked up my cell phone, and dialled. Ralph picked up on the other end. "I am on my way to the hospital to have an abortion right now, and the kid is yours. I thought that you should know," I told him. I remember there being a deadly silence on the other end. Apparently, he had no idea what to say, and so with that, I said goodbye and hung up. When Mandy got back to the car, I told her that I had called him. And off we went.

When we got there, this really, really nice nurse looked after me. She had real compassion, and seemed to truly care about me. I wish to this day, that I could remember her name, because I have always wanted to thank the woman. I knew and had been told that when they perform these abortions, the patient is left coherent, and knows what is going on. I cried, and pleaded with the nurse to please, please, please, knock me out with something. I told her that there is no way that I can do this, and go through with it consciously. She told me that she would be there with me, and do what she could to help. She was not allowed to "knock me out" however. I do not know why, or how I did it, but she complied. The next thing I knew, I was waking up in the recovery room. I missed the whole thing, and never in my life, have I been more thankful.

So then, that was that...painful part over. I have always known deep down inside that the little person that was inside me, was a little boy. It was only about a month ago, that I took the time to say goodbye to him. I have never been able to really recognize what I had done, and laying in my hammock on my patio one sunny day, he came before me. I was glad.

Okay, so now, another thing has just popped back into my head, and I do not think I have told you this part yet. I know it was just after Ralph and I had first split up, but were still "on and off." I had been for a pap smear once in a while probably, but not regularly. My doctor called me back in one day, after having run my tests, and sat me down. He explained that over the last couple of years, my tests had come back pretty much okay, but there was something amiss. It was small and insignificant, but the fact that it had shown up more than once or twice, led him to err on the side of caution. I was then sent for a biopsy, and I was pretty scared. Ralph had been kind enough to come with me, and had given me a ride to the hospital. A few weeks later, my biopsy results came back, and sure enough, it was determined that I had cervical cancer. Cancer runs in my family on my mother's side, both her sister and my Grandma have died of cancer. Her brother died from other causes, and her father, from a gunshot in the war. My Grandfather had come home to die in his bed.

I was thankful to have Ralph by my side, and did not really want to worry any of my friends and family with it at the time. He took me back in for the "laser surgery" procedure, they had scheduled. First, I had to meet with the specialist that would do the surgery. I will never forget the raw excitement this old English doctor portrayed, as I walked into his office. He greeted me, and shook my hand as though I were a celebrity for Gosh's sake. He sat me down in a chair, and sat across his big desk, animatedly excited. "Let me explain," he said, "why I am so excited." It turned out as he explained to me, that I was "out of the text books." He told me how he had discussed my case with many old timers and young doctors alike, and had checked all resources and medical journals. Never, ever, ever, had anyone seen, or documented, the same location where the cancer was found. He proceeded to draw me a bunch of pictures, showing me where the cervical cancers are usually found, and where mine was located. It was all French to me, but will always stay in my mind, due to his excitement.

And so, they gave me another appointment for the actual procedure. They showed Ralph and I a video of what it was they were going to do to me exactly. I wished they had not have shown me, because it just made me more nervous. What they do is locate the tumour, and go over and over it with a laser beam, in effect burning it off. Then came another "moment in time," that will always stick with me, as the nurse and I rode up together in an elevator. I asked how long it would take, and she informed me that the majority of surgeries were over within two minutes. I had also been informed that the surgeon (that old guy) does not believe in anaesthetics and although doctors knocked most people out, he would provide only a local anaesthetic. That's just how he did things, and don't worry, I was told.

I was brought into the operating room, and as I lay there waiting, I felt strange, and scared. The next thing I knew, in the door he comes, barely greets me, goes straight to my lower parts, and this is the next thing that I heard. "Well, this is a big one! It will take at least ten minutes." My heart sank, and then I felt the searing pain. I could actually feel how the laser beam went over and over and over the same spot. It was a stinging, burning sensation, and I tried and tried to tune out what was really going on. Until I smelled the smell of burning flesh. I don't know if it was "in my head," but now it hurt even more. It was an awful procedure, as I remember it, and something I would not recommend without anaesthetics. It worked though, and I have remained cancer free for all these years.

Okay, so now we've made it past some more unpleasantries in the life of Petra Hoffmann. Lucky for you, it doesn't end here, and I already have a second book in mind. There is too much in my life that keeps happening, and so it will not fit into just one book!

Now what should we discuss next? Oh, I know. I had made a plan to move to my hometown when I discovered that Australia was out of the question. By this time, thankfully, Kaytlin was going to Gabriola Island. Her grandparents on her dad's side, Pete and Marcella, had bought some "swampland" there, many years prior. When they sold their home in Surrey, and then sold the apartment they lived in for a couple of years, they decided to sell the swampland also, and buy something on the island. Gabriola Island is a twenty minute ferry ride from the main island. From Vancouver, it translates into a five hour trip, two hours on one ferry and then a drive, and then a wait (runs once an hour) to Gabriola on another ferry.

Kaytlin was to spend a few weeks at her grandparent's house, and the timing was perfect. I figured, that I would first get a job in town, and then look for a place, while she was gone. And with that I began my job at a bar in Point Roberts. Point Roberts is a little piece of the United States, that can be gotten to either by ocean, or through my home town of Tsawwassen. It was a nightmare to get to work however, and with my current drug addiction plus no car, not easy. It took me three buses to get to the border. There I had to call the bar and someone usually picked me up. I don't even remember how long the whole trip there took, but it was several hours. Although the owner, Neil, was very abusive to his staff, I loved working there. He wasn't around much anyway. The money was alright, with the tips were good. We also had a pull tab bar, which I loved working at.

Finally, I met someone who lived near me, and so when they were on shift, I could get a ride to or from work once in a while. I literally worked my butt off at the Breakers. It was right on the beach. Most times, I would already be on the phone with my dealer, while I was still on route home. I had timed it so that he and I would arrive at my place about the same time, so I would not have to wait. Then I'd be up for most of the night, and go to work the next day, tired as hell. It soon really started to show on me...the lack of sleep, the lack of self maintenance, and the weight loss. Whenever I see someone today that looks like I did then, I know. People even began asking if I was okay?

I spoke to Kaytlin on the phone everyday, and missed her like crazy, but at the same time, I was glad that she did not see me like this. There was one night in particular that stands out. I had called at the usual time, and Kaytlin said to me, "Mommy, Gabriola Island is paradise, mommy. You should see it." "I will, baby," I said, "but I have to use my time off to look for a place here, like we planned, remember?" "I do, she said, "but, Mommy, it would be my dream come true to move to Gabriola Island." Those were the exact words she used, I remember it so vividly. I stopped, and thought for a moment. "Do you really mean that?" I queried. "Yes, it would be my dream come true," she said again. "Alright," I replied, "I have two days off this week, and I will come out there. I promise that I will come with an open mind, and if I love it as much as you, we will discuss it further. Is that fair?" Excitedly she agreed, and then we said good night, and she put her Nana on the phone, and we made the plans.

And so, a few days later, I headed to Gabriola Island for the first time. The trip there was beautiful, as I took one ferry across our incredible ocean waters, on a gorgeous sunny summer day! My father in law took Kaytlin and I around the island to go and look at some rentals. I'm not sure if we can count the first place we looked at, because it was a house in the trees. A tiny little one bedroom perched amongst the branches. "Creative," I thought, "but not for us." The second place we looked at, I fell in love with instantly. It was a two year old beautiful house which sat perched upon a man built hill, atop a long winding driveway. The house itself was to die for. It was a one bedroom, in the back, along with a small closet laundry room, then down the hall, opening up into a bright, big kitchen on your left, and straight ahead, was a full wall of picture windows that opened up into the living room. On the left again was a bright dining room, with another sliding door onto a fair sized wrap around patio.

Now, come with me through the living room, which by the way had a thirty foot ceiling, and more picture windows, up high. Through the living room, and up another staircase on your right, and at the top of the railing, sat a huge loft, in the shape of an upside down V. It also had 2 other windows looking over the back of the house, which was forested. The loft would be my bedroom, and I had never been in a brighter, more beautiful home. I stood against the loft railing and looked straight ahead of me, and out the picture windows.

Below the hill on which the house sat, there was a two acre meadow, with a fenced off garden running along the left side by the road, and in the middle of it all, there was a duck pond. I was sold...I did not need to see anything else, for it all paled in comparison. As we continued our journey around the island, I fell more and more in love. There was a feeling of magic in the air, pristine, barely touched, wilderness all around. My Kaytlin was right! Gabriola Island was a literal paradise, and when I left again the next day, it was with relief and pure joy in my heart. I think I had found our new home. How could this be wrong? "Not to mention," I thought, "I would be getting away from all the drugs in the city." I was sure that one could not get drugs on an island such as this, and it would keep me safe from them forever. I again, (for the first time in a long time) now had something to look forward to.

I came back to Surrey, gave notice at my job, and worked for another few weeks. Of course, I also gave notice at the dark dingy hell hole I lived in. Thank Gosh, I had not unpacked anything we didn't use daily, so there was not too much to do. I made arrangements to rent a truck, and off I went. The only thing that kind of put a damper on my arrival, was the fact that Jane and her boyfriend Arnell, had beat me there. They were actually sitting on my new property waiting for me to arrive. Not only that, but they had already been all over the island, looking at property for themselves. "Oh my Gosh," I thought, "that is all I need, for Jane to follow me to Gabe and fuck it all up somehow." I feel in my heart that she has always been jealous of me, (and I may be wrong). I always had a lot of friends, and Jane could not hold on to a friend (except for me).

Not very often have I been able to get her to come out and do things together with my other friends. Whenever I did, it still stands out in my mind. One time, for example, I took her with me to meet about eight others at a neighbourhood pub. They were all really close friends, so of course they gave me their opinion. The only reason being of course, that she had put me down a lot, throughout the couple of hours we spent with them. It has always been the consensus, after meeting her, that she is jealous of me. I suppose that I was just used to it. My mother always puts me down in front of my friends as well.

Anyways, I did not want her on my island with me. This was to be MY home, and I knew that she would ruin it for us. The fact that they were looking at property and restaurants to buy scared me. So, other than that, it was a great arrival, and in all fairness, it was nice to see familiar faces in an unfamiliar land. Not to mention have a few "Welcome to our new Home" drinks with Jane. After all, she is about the biggest alcoholic, addict I know. She cannot live without a drink in her hand, and pharmaceuticals down her throat. Every time she and I have had a falling out, it becomes clear to me that the only reason she wants me in her life is to party with. We sure have had some fun times, and scary ones too.

I know I am getting off topic here again, but I just remembered some stuff I had forgotten to tell you about. I don't know how far the news from Vancouver spreads around the Globe, or where you are right now. There was a big bust that went down here a few years ago, and is still in the public's eye and on the local news, all the time.

One day I got a call from my dad, and he said to me, "You remember telling me about that pig farm you've partied at before?' "Sure," I said, "what about it?" "Well, that is the pig farmer they just arrested for killing all those girls." It had made front page headlines for days now. "No, Dad," I said, "the place I went to was called "Piggy's Palace." I had been there at least five to seven times, for parties on Thanksgiving and the such. "That's right," he said, "and the pig farmer, Robert Pickton, is the one up on charges." Suddenly it all played back through my head. A good friend of mine, Guy, had taken me there the first time, and I was introduced to a couple of guys that were at the door. One of them was Robert himself, gumboots and all. As it all came back to me now, I recalled recoiling from his handshake, and turning the other way to talk to someone. The guy was so dirty looking, and something about him just creeped me out. Instinct...thank Gosh I have always had a very strong instinct. The same thing which I honed in Kaytlin. I believe that society tries to breed it out of us, and I wanted my daughter to make sure that she always followed her gut, and so I taught her from a very young age, how.

It has literally saved her...one time in particular. Her aunt was baby sitting and wanted to leave her alone with her boyfriend. Kaytlin was five years old and thought I would be mad, because she didn't "listen to an adult." She refused to be left alone with him, and finally her aunt conceded and took her to where she was going. "That," I explained, "is the gut feeling, that warns you of danger, and I am so very proud of you for listening to that." "You did the right thing, Kaytlin, and I will never be mad at you for that," I explained when she told me what had happened. It turned out years later, that same man was arrested for paedophile activities in Nanaimo. He was a known paedophile! So, there, you see, how close we sometimes come in life? It still plays on my mind that I ate the turkey there on Thanksgiving, and although I did not eat any pig, it haunts me. You see, if you have heard of the case...he fed the remains of the women he killed to the pigs!

# Chapter 9 – Gabriola Island

Sorry for steering you all off course again...there are so many tales that won't fit in this book. But, without further ado, our new life on Gabriola Island begins!

Jane and Arnell went back home after the long weekend...and KK and I found ourselves alone at last. What a beautiful house, and what a beautiful yard, and what a beautiful island! Shitty thing was, I had no car, and I knew not one soul, other than my mother and father in law. Oh, also my sister in law lived on Gabe with her three girls. Wanda is a super addict. She will do whatever she can get her hands on, and so I have tried through trial and error not to spend too much time with her. But, believe it or not, it was Gabriola Days the following weekend, and so we made plans to go out together. First, we would take the girls to the community hall for a dinner and dance, and then the plan was to drop them all off with "Nana and Grumps," and party on! Sounded like fun to this girl, "what better way to meet people," I thought. And, ohhhhh, what a night it turned out to be. Haha, I will never forget most of it.

I had begun to drink lemon drops, which were introduced to me at an annual lobster fest, by a good friend of mine. I in turn was nice enough to introduce the island to them. You know how you do a shot of tequila, but first you lick the salt from the curve of your hand between your thumb and forefinger? So, salt, shot, and then a bite of lime? Most of you have done that, I'm sure? If not, it is a must try. Anyways, a "lemon drop is "sugar, shot of Vodka, and (you guessed it) lemon! With this the party began. We had the booze in the car, and simply couldn't wait to get started. It did not take much encouragement before we left the girls with Nana and Grumps, and headed out to the car to do shots. The community hall party went really well...we danced fervently (as you can imagine) with the girls, and everyone had a good time. Until, Wanda came back in.

She had gone out to the car to smoke a joint, and it was her third or fourth trip out. Well, I guess that since it was a family affair, some onlookers had taken it upon themselves to call the cops on her. And the cops were waiting by her car when she had come back out. Luckily, the last time I had gone out to do a shot with her, Wanda had told me that she did not trust her daughter and her daughter's friends. She told me to take the vodka bottle in with me. So, I had it stashed in my purse. Lucky for Wanda, as they went through the car, and found the sugar and the lemon remains, but no booze! She admitted to smoking a joint, and denied anything else, and they let her go. But they had asked that she leave the hall. It was almost over anyway, and so we rounded up the kids, and sent them home with their grandparents.

We went back up to Wanda's place to change, and from there we went to the bar. There are actually three bars on the island. Gabriola Island is about 30 miles long, and 15 miles wide. There is North Road and South Road, and they meet again in a circle. By car it is about 45 minutes around the whole island, and it is breathtaking. South Road goes by some homes, then a golf course with a lake, and then breathtaking ocean views. North Road is well known for it's "tree tunnel." The trees grow along the road and envelope it at their height. You should see it at Halloween time, when the residents come and put their pumpkins in throughout the tunnel. I'll tell you more about the island later though, as I am getting off course again.

We stayed at the bar for a while and met a few people there. "Everyone is so nice, and I feel completely welcome and at home here," I thought. We ended up meeting whom I thought to be a very good looking guy named Danny. But before I could get to know him better, Wanda whisked me off to another party she had been invited to. We were getting really smashed by now, or at least I know I was. So, off to the party we went. It was a house party, and there were people everywhere. I met a few of them, and then I spotted him in the kitchen. The same good looking guy I had met at the bar. So, off to the kitchen Petra went, of course. We got into a deep conversation, and he told me so much about my new home. I'm not sure if I heard much of what he said, but I do recall introducing him to lemon drops.

And then...shit...my mouth starts to water. Shit, you know the feeling just before you are about to puke? I did not even have a chance to excuse myself, as I raced outside, my hand covering my mouth. As I got out the front door, there was Wanda, surrounded by a large group of people. As I ran past, she tried to stop me to make introductions. I shook myself loose, and made it about three more steps, and then I had to let her rip. Yup...right in front of them all. "Hello," I said sheepishly, "how embarrassing. I am Wanda's sister in law." All I remember after that is wanting to get the hell out of there. I was so embarrassed. And so, folks, that ends the tale of my first party on Gabriola Island.

Okay, so we are now at the end of September of the year 2000. Gray had wanted to live to see the new era. He didn't make it quite that far, but he made it three and a half years past his initial diagnosis, and that, given the odds, was a miracle. And, he was right...had he died when KK was five years old rather than eight, she would not have remembered him so vividly. Anyways, I sure missed him. I missed picking up the phone either at random, or when I needed to talk about something, and having Gray to talk to about it. He never did judge. He had to have known that I was having drug issues, when he died, and my promise to him to be the best mother I could be, was understood only by him. His mother never got it, and we have had a few disagreements about what I said to Grayson on his deathbed. I cannot convince her that she heard wrong, and I know in my heart that Gray knew that I was doing my best.

One promise I made to myself, was that if ever I thought that our daughter would be better off under someone else's care, I would have done whatever would be best for her. Gray is one of the few people who deeply knows my inner spirit. I'm not sure if that makes any sense. I always have a big mouth, and I tell people about my life, but there are some things I keep guarded. Only love can get through that, true love, not misguided love. Ralph for example has never known me as deeply as Gray did. Nor did Dennis. Most likely because they didn't know how to truly love.

So, then, at Capon, which I call the house, for it was on Capon Drive, just off south road, not too far from the "tree tunnel." At Capon I unpacked. I found it very difficult there though, because I was on the "other side of the island." You see, all the stores and most of the population were on the ferry side of the island. On my side there was only a pub and marina, and a lot of farm land. When I first had arrived and began asking around for work, I met Clarke. There is a book out about his family being the original pirates who stopped everyone coming in to the island. He owns the golf course, and a lot of property on Gabriola. Basically he owns a lot of the island. Anyways, this eccentric character, had the audacity to offer me a job shearing sheep. I had never heard anything so ludicrous before, and looked at him aghast. "Do I look like a sheep shearer to you?" I sputtered. He laughed so hard, and has liked me ever since. Not enough to offer me any other work though, come to think of it!

Work, on a little island, the population of which was about 4,000 when I first moved there, was difficult to find. It was difficult at the house, because I could not even afford to get a phone hooked up at first. I ran my cell phone over the limit, and eventually got cut off. The hardest thing was, that being winter, (and we got a lot of snow there) if I needed milk or something, I could not call and tell anyone. Pete and Marcella did come by and check on us once or twice a week, but there was no way to let them know what we needed. "I have to do something," I thought. I do not recall who I met or how...oh, yes, it just came to me. Of course I had now enrolled Kaytlin in school, which was also on the other end of the island...(what wasn't?) I figured that she needed something or someone to help her through the loss. I asked around, and came across a group called Rainbows, set up for children that had suffered loss either through divorce, or death. It was a great group run by some extremely caring girls, and I think it was good for KK. It was there that I ended up volunteering, at the centre that held this group. It was called People Living for a Healthier Community, now called the Gathering Place. I went in, I think twice a week, and worked in the office. I loved it, but needed to have an income.

Ultimately it was not long before I began to meet people. Let's not forget here, (for I could not) the drug habit with which I had arrived. I really wanted to get high, and before long, I asked a new friend of mine Lionel where I could score. He led me to the "pink house." Yes...go figure...another "pink house!" Andy, the renter of the house was obviously well known on the island. Everyone knew him, and he had the biggest best parties, all the time. For example, every Easter weekend, we would hide beer rather than eggs, and another three day party would be born. I soon discovered that on Gabiola Island, every day is a party, and there is a party every night. People here are "on island time," and rarely does anyone show up on time for a meeting. I met most of the island party animals and residents at the first "pink house" party I attended. Things were off and running after that. I was in party heaven. There was a ton of the white stuff all around, and the bathrooms, bedrooms, and dining rooms were filled with mirrors, and straws.

I still found it difficult however, to get crack cocaine, or to get out of the door and not have to share it with others. I was only able to do it once, (because he was too scared to send it twice) but I convinced Mack, that realtor friend of mine, to mail me some already cooked. I will never forget the day it arrived in the mail, and my mother in law had given me a ride to the mailbox. By the way, my mailbox was down at the end of Capon, left on North road, and then another couple of country blocks down the road. I tell you, there is no place darker than Gabe at night, with no street lighting.

So, getting back to my little package in the mail. I ran upstairs to my loft, while KK and Nana made some tea in the kitchen. Obviously, she wasn't leaving any time soon. My fingers were shaking so hard in anticipation of what I knew would be in there. Sure enough, there was a light brown coloured square of crack. I could not wait to try it. I shook so hard, as I positioned the screen I kept in my room to hide what I was doing. I pulled out my home-made pipe, shaking even harder now, knowing I could so easily get caught. I broke off a little hoot and threw it in the pipe. Oh...that first hit. I hope they didn't hear the lighter, but I would pretend I was having a cigarette, for I was a smoker after all. I sat there a moment, and let the rush wash over me. "Pretty good stuff," I thought, "now how am I going to act straight?" I realized again that I should never do this shit while KK was around and especially awake. What was I thinking? And then the guilt began to wash over me.

"How am I going to get rid of Marcella, so I can do more," I thought, as I came down the stairs. "What took you so long up there?" Marcella asked, as I came down the stairs. "Oh, just reading a letter a friend sent me," I said, hoping that she wouldn't notice that I was all jittery. I then declined the cup of tea offered, laid on the couch and pretended that I had a migraine, so she would go away. It seemed like forever before Marcella finally left, and I could tell KK that I was going to go lay down in my room. She was pretty much on her own for the rest of the day, as I laid there feigning a headache. I prayed that she would not come up the stairs, every time I got up and snuck another hoot, hiding the stuff and the pipe again every time. It all seems so cheap and sorted, and ugly to me, looking back on it all now. I really was being a terrible mother, and would not be able to live with myself, if my daughter knew of my problem.

Lionel spent our first Christmas on Gabriola with us, and it was pretty good. He was the first guy I met, and befriended. I think my parents came to the island and spent some time with us, just after Christmas. They fell in love with Gabriola as soon as they arrived, as had I. I didn't have a lot of money, and racked my brain trying to find a solution. I had a good idea, and got Lionel to take me to the SPCA in Nanaimo, a twenty minute ferry ride away. There I fell in love with a little black and white ball of fluff. It was a border collie, terrier cross. I had no idea how high maintenance these little souls would be. And so, when Christmas eve arrived, I went back to town earlier that day and picked up the dog. Lionel and I came up with a great idea. We took a big cardboard box, and wrapped it in Xmas paper, leaving a hole to peak though in the back, so the puppy didn't freak out. Then we called KK out of her room, where I had asked her to wait while Santa came and dropped off her gifts.

I know that a puppy was the last thing she expected, because I had told her "no" so many times before. Her eyes opened wide, when she approached the box slowly, and it began to move across the floor. Then she saw the little face peeking out of the hole, and I had one happy little girl for Xmas 2000!

Next, I met Tabatha. Tabatha was the head bartender at the pub next to the ferry terminal, the White Hart. We hit it off pretty much right away. I realized soon enough that some nights (as in all bars) it gets pretty boring, and that bartenders love company. She and I began hanging out, and she was having a tryst with a fellow by the name of Jeff. His best friend was Danny. Before long, the four of us started hanging out together, and since I was the only one who had the kid at home, we usually ended up at my place. I missed Ralph like crazy and I had never, ever had any sort of closure with Ethan, whom I knew I loved, but believed was married. I had lost my best friend, and father to my daughter, and my heart was now closed. Closed as closed could get.

I missed my drugs, I missed my life style, fucked up as it had been. I missed my life as it was, and I needed something. I am not rightly sure how things progressed or in what order, but the four of us began sleeping together, at my place, in my loft. I had never done anything like this sexually before, and now in hindsight, I realize that it became my new drug. There were no strings, there was no jealousy, nothing, because my heart was not involved. Tabatha and Jeff were an item for a couple of years, and for them it created a facet to their relationship they needed, for whatever reasons. Danny and I just had great sex, and other than that, there were no ties. We were free to do as we pleased. Whenever Kaytlin was gone, it was pretty much a given that we spend those days together at my house, and when she was home, they would leave once in while.

I suppose the only drawback to the situation, was that after a while, I felt used. I fed them, they would use all my toiletries, sometimes do their laundry, and after a while I felt it in my pocketbook. Tabatha often pissed me off because she always expected a ride home or to work. The guilt that riddled me in my clear moments was unthinkable, and so as if on auto pilot, my life continued. Before long, I had a job at Silva Bay, a nearby marina, on my side of the island. Soon after I had a job doing census for the government. And why not do some taxes on the side to round it all out?

I mentioned that I was giving Tabatha and the others rides, and yes, after having received a couple of pay checks, I had invested in a really nice blue Daytona. It was a nice looking vehicle. Kaytlin's friends all thought it pretty cool. Oh, Gosh, here we go again about that Jane "friend" of mine. I had come from the island to visit with Jane and the boys, upon their invitation. I took this opportunity to look for a new vehicle to purchase. After just two days there however, I began to feel as though I were imposing to the highest degree. I had no car to get around in, and so we were at her mercy. Arnell and Jane were living together, and his brother owned the Daytona, and was selling it.

Long story short, I had to get the hell out of there. Kaytlin and I were left hungry because no one really fed us, and I was not comfortable enough to make us anything myself. Jane was kind of in and out doing whatever she was doing, so I would take that opportunity to make us a quick sandwich or something. It felt horrible to be there, and I needed to leave and quickly. I had not ever felt so very unwelcome anywhere in my life before. But Jane had a way of doing that to me, and it was not the first time. She would invite me to stay, and then make me feel like I was a burden, and was overstaying my welcome. It is no wonder that she was unable to make and keep friends, and I suppose that is why I hung in so long. I always felt sorry for her, knowing that Dotty and I were her only real friends. Dotty, by the way is no longer a part of Jane's world now anymore either. Hasn't been in many years. And so, I bought the first car I looked at, Arnell's brother's car, just so I could get Kaytlin and I the hell out of there.

The next person that came into my life on Gabriola Island was a young girl twenty years my junior whom I had met at Andy Swallow's party, (at the pink house.) I remember that she told me the same thing that others have said to me, and that is that she tried not to like me, but could not help herself. My sister in law had told me that same thing one day. Tabatha, Jeff and Danny kind of faded into the background, as things had kind of run their course, as most of these things do. Alison and I became really close friends. Kaytlin really liked her too, and the best part was that Alison had an apartment right at Silva Bay, because she worked there also. It worked out great for me, because she was able to look after Kaytlin when I worked, and I could just pop over for my breaks, and spend more time with KK that way.

Alison was in party mode. I worked three jobs, and I will never figure out exactly how I did it, but I began partying and pulling "all nighters" right along with her. On Gabriola Island, ladies and gentlemen, boys and girls, there is a party every single night of the week. They are in bars, they are in homes, they are in yards, they are in fields, and they are on the beach. What I love most about "home" is that there is so much musical talent there. I have always loved music, and it has brought me back from the edge of the abyss more that once. As a matter of fact, I know almost all the words to every song ever recorded. It is not something that I even realized I did, until my daughter looked at me in wonder in the car one day, where I always sing along at the top of my lungs, and said "Mommy, how do you know the words to every single song?" I tell you here and now, that had Gosh given Petra a voice, I would have loved nothing more than to sing for my supper! There is nothing I love more. But alas, I soon found out in school, (for I was in every choir group they had) that I cannot carry a tune.

I will never, ever forget what it was like to have such incredible talent and love of music, in my very own living room, or around my very own fire-pit, in mine or in my neighbours' yards. I will never forget the talent in the bars, and on the beaches, and in the parks. It touches your soul in such an intense way that it brings tears to my eyes even now.

The only frustrating part is that with all the talent on Gabe, (and having a great ear for music) one cannot convince these island loving people to ever leave in order to perform out in the world. I recall a few years later, I befriended Chastity, whose family is so musical. Chastity was over at my place one day when a call came in for her. I overheard the whole thing. It was a casting call for one of those shows that goes around the whole world, a massive musical group that performs a tribute to major musicians. They do a new one every year. I could not believe my ears when Chas turned down this huge opportunity. She was a shoe-in, they had called her, and she said "No, thank you," without blinking an eye. How many people get that sort of opportunity? No one has every given me a break in my entire life, and I just found it so unfathomable that others could pass one over so easily. Almost as though it had never even happened. I'm sure that I still think about it more, than Chastity does.

Anyways, as I mentioned, I managed to maintain three jobs for a while. I worked at the bar, usually out on the open air patio overlooking the cove and marina, and oh, what a setting! My second job was doing taxes and bookkeeping, for I had started up my own business, having worked for the government for so long. My third job, which I crazily took on was working for Census Canada. It was the hardest two months of my life. I found homes up in trees, with power in. I had to cliff climb and bush whack to find some of these "residences." There are a lot of people on the gulf islands, I soon learned who did not want to be discovered. It is the law which says that one must post the house number on your home, so they would post it on the back door. Knowing this, we were provided city maps, that depicted most of the hidden properties, but if no one was home, and you had to go back again, good luck finding it. It became somewhat confusing to be sure.

I was sitting outside of the White Hart pub with a friend early one Saturday morning, after having partied all night the evening before. I'd been having a leisurely cup of coffee, when I got a call on my cell. It was my supervisor, asking if I had read the morning paper. "No, why?" I hesitantly asked. "Because you are in it," he said. He did not sound impressed, so I had to get the paper. Sure enough there it was, in the "Snarls" column of all places. Well, actually it was called the “Smiles and Snarls,” but this was a definite snarl. It read as follows: “Thank you to the Census worker who ran into our deer gate and took off!” “Oh, shit,” I laughed with my friend. I had become the U-turn Queen of Gabriola, trying to find these stinking addresses. I remembered this one very well. The sun had been right in my eyes as I pulled into a driveway. The “chicken coop mesh,” which they called their “deer gate” was entirely transparent, absolutely invisible to the human eye. I hit it, pulled back, and recall seeing the imprint of my car in the “fence.” There, was, however a couple of huge German Sheppard dogs that viciously bore down on me. I left the Census forms, hanging on the fence by the mail box. I mean, there was no way with those dogs I was going in. Hello!?

One night I had a very vivid dream. I have a lot of vivid dreams. It is and was, and always will be a most poignant part of my life. Sorry to be getting off track again, but you should be used to it by now. Lol Once upon a time, before Gray died, I had what up until today has been the most intense, vivid dream I have ever had. We were driving along, Gray at the wheel, in a station wagon of all things. I hate station wagons. Everything seemed okay, and suddenly a feeling came upon me, greater and more powerful than anything that I had ever felt. I knew beyond a shadow of a doubt that we were about to crash and that one of us had to die. I looked over at him, and he knew also. I knew that too. The next thing you know, we were looking at each other, then straight ahead, and a huge argument ensued. We were fighting over who was going to be the one to die. I had no doubt that I would die for him, quite happily almost. But he wasn’t in agreement.

He told me that he had to die, that he knew that he would be the one. I screamed, I pleaded, I begged, to let me be the one. “I know that it is you, who is the better parent. I know that you will do a better job with our daughter, than I could ever even dream to do,” I pleaded. Grayson, in my mind then, and in the dream, and even now, and forever, in my opinion was the best dad to his children that I have ever seen. He lived and breathed for them. He did everything for them. I handpicked that man. He was the one who had to stay, not me. But, no matter how hard I pleaded, I was not the one to win this argument. I didn’t need to see the crash, I knew then that it was Gray who would die. Premonition...perhaps?

So, then, back to my job at Silva Bay. I could tell that the owner and especially his wife did not like me much. What was worse is that he was really abusive. He treated his staff like lowly slaves, always telling us to move faster, move better, do more. Nothing was ever good enough for this pompous French ass hole. I began having visions of catching Gilles and his giant walkie talkie on one of the docks and pushing the bastard over the edge, wearing nothing but some lovely cement shoes. It has always been hard for me to bite my tongue, but I did. I lasted there for about three months, and then, out of the blue, for no apparent reason, Gilles called me over after my shift one day, and told me that I was being let go. I think he said I was too slow, although I was always the one covering for the others when they got caught behind. I had not ever in my life been "fired" off a job before. I did not take it very well, and must have cried for a week solid. That, of course turned into more partying and drugs, in an attempt to once again numb the pain. I could not believe that I had moved here to get away from drugs, and had run right into the lap.

Teresa lived just up the road from me, and she and I started using together, along with her boyfriend, Denny. At this time, we still had to go to Nanaimo to score most of the time. The dealers on the island were not at my disposal, and always on their own schedule, or out altogether. When I got that Daytona, I used to race to that last ferry, and made it clear across the island in 18 minutes flat a couple of times. That, my friends, was really risking it, because the island is overrun with little brown tailed deer, and I was lucky that one never jumped out at the wrong time. When it is the last boat for the night though, and you have just run out, you do what you have to do to get there.

Again, I tried to pull myself back up somehow. There was no work to be had on the island, census had finished, and I ended up about $1,000 short on my pay. Tax season was over, and I needed to get another job. And, so, I applied for one in Nanaimo, at a call centre for Bell in the states. It became a really, really, long day, and with the almost daily drug use now, I was getting worn out. My job was an eight hour a day job, but the commute to Nanaimo from the farthest side of the island was another four to seven more hours. I would take the first ferry out, which was usually overloaded, so you had to get there an hour early. It took at least a half hour to get to the ferry. Then the twenty five minute drive on the other side to work. Coming back, in rush hour presented more overloaded ferries, and sometimes you had to wait another two hours, since they only run once an hour each way. Then I would have to drive up the other side of the island, where KK's grandparents lived, who babysat for me. Oh, yes, wait, first I had to drop her off there in the morning. That was another half hour each way. All in all, it was a fourteen to sixteen hour day! I thought that if I were to move to the other side of the island, I could shave off some of this time, and save some money on rent. My place was very expensive for the island.

Now, I may or may not have mentioned earlier, that I had a lot of company from the mainland, and my parents had come out several times, and stayed with us. They fell in love with Gabriola, and unfortunately decided to sell their dream house in Tsawwassen. This was the same year that my mother retired from the high school in which she worked. My dad then moved them both to my island, and I knew that this paradise had now come to an end for me somehow. The island was way too small for my fucked up family.

Anyways, my dad bought the home they moved into, and also a property with a small one bedroom cabin on it, as well as a couple of building lots. He had taken on a new business partner, an investor, a woman he had known for years, and now began to "work" very closely with. The cabin had no running water or kitchen sink at all. The shower and washer/dryer and a deep laundry sink were in a separate building. He offered to rent me the cabin for $300 or $350 (not sure which) per month, which cut my bills in more than half. I really needed to get back on my feet, and so I took it. So, sure, I shaved about an hour commute off of my day. But since there was also no heat (other than a tiny wood stove) and it was getting to be winter again, I had to chop wood myself. Then I had to load the wood stove before work, and again, as soon as we got back late at night. It was like camping every single day, and not so bad until the summer was over. All my dishes had to be carried back and forth, to the out building, and I broke a lot of them. I had to do the dishes in the deep laundry sink, and carry water to cook with.

The good news was that I was too busy and too tired with all the extra work, that I did not use a lot of crack at the cabin. Besides, it was harder to hide with it. The few times I did get some there, I would hide in the outbuilding, and sit on the toilet (the only seat in the house), and tweak out, shaking after every hoot, figuring I was going to get caught. All the sounds (when you smoke this stuff) become amplified, so with the deer and the raccoon just outside the door, it was a trip alright. I wonder often, how it is that us addicts find that enjoyable in our messed up thinking, enough so as to purchase more.

The part of our memories which get access when we yearn for the drug, is the part that does that first or second hit. There is a certain protective warmth, almost like the arms of an angel, that envelopes and surrounds you so completely, that it is sometimes better than an orgasm. You just don't allow yourself to remember the rest. The shaking, and the amplification of all sounds, and sights, and imaginings. The tenseness in ones entire body, all muscles on constant alert, feeling as though your heart is about to explode, or perhaps your brain will go first? How difficult to explain why us addicts do this, or why. I have found in my personal experience that it is mostly hurt and pain at first that drives our addictions, and then it just becomes boredom. Then, when you begin to isolate yourself, like I was doing and had been doing for so long now, the boredom naturally grows, and so does ones desire to escape it. Especially on an island in the winter, when it is so very easy to isolate.

I have to keep reminding myself of the pain, and the negatives that surround drug addiction. I do not ever want to forget what I have done in the past to get clean. The detoxification, the mind games, the horror of having to face yourself in the mirror when you become straight, the horror of facing others straight. How do you act, what do you say? Do they all know? Can they see it? Can they feel it? Are they thinking it? You see, it you do not change your circle, you cannot become sober, they will bring you back down. Addicts are afraid of being addicts all alone.

So then, the next few months were extremely difficult. I was finding it hard not to use, but falling into bed most nights out of pure exhaustion helped. I needed to get out of there though. I no longer liked "camping every day." My dad did nothing to help make the living arrangements better. For example, I was sleeping on the floor in the living room, and there was a half inch gap under the door, that would blow right in on me. I begged him to come over and fix it, but it was more important for him to put shelving in his laundry room at their place than to help us in any way. I made sure that his rent was always paid, and when I did finally move, Gray's family came to help me clean as well. We washed every wall, so that nothing could be said about the way I left his cabin.

While at the cabin, I had given a friend of mine a ride to Nanaimo one day, with his dog named Sally. As we drove, he told me that he was moving back east to look after his ailing parents, and that he could only afford to take his old dog. Since this one was new and he was not really attached, he was going to have to board her until (if ever) he could afford to fly her out. "I would love to find her a new home," he said. As he told the story, I kept looking back at Sally in the back seat, and I swear she knew what he was talking about. I have never seen such a sad looking face. And she was beautiful. Sally was about one and a half at this time, and she was a lab, husky, wolf, cross. She looked just like a golden lab retriever, only slimmer, with a bit longer face, and a bit bushier tail, in which one could see the wolf markings. Red nose. Before I knew it had even come out of my mouth, as I looked back one more time, I heard myself saying, "I want her." He looked at me stunned. We agreed after a bit of negotiation, that he would put his trip off for a few more days, and come back to my place with Sally. I would see if Kaytlin, Sally, and I clicked, and at the end of a week, either give her back, or hopefully keep her.

Sally, it turned out, was a very special spirit, and Kaytlin and I became attached almost immediately. I have not to this day, come across a better, kinder, more gentle animal, whom everybody fell in love with. I am not kidding, she was the best. All Sally ever wanted was to be with me, after that. She loved car rides more than anything in the world. If I even thought to myself, that I was going to go somewhere, she would read my mind, and go and wait by the car, in case I left her behind. Whenever I was at work, or out without her, she would try to break away. My neighbour was kind enough to make her a huge run the width of the yard, which was about three properties wide. Sometimes though, she would still get away. Whenever she did, she would go to the mall...always towards the lights and sounds.

There were three occasions when people on the island kept her overnight, just so they could spend some time with her, while I would look for her all night. Everyone that brought her back, begged to keep her. Everywhere we went, people told me that if I ever got rid of her, they wanted her. She was a special spirit, I tell you. I have never loved an animal more than I love my Silly Sally, as I called her.

Sally hated it when I got high. That is always when she would act up, and take off somewhere, often returning, after having rolled in otter shit at the beach. She did it on purpose. Otter shit is like tar, it sticks to their coat, and is very difficult to remove. And boy, does it smell something awful! Sally loved the water more than anything. You could take her to the beach and throw the stick in the ocean all day long. When you got tired, she would take the stick to anyone on the beach to have them throw it for her. I could take her anywhere, even to Nanaimo, and never on a leash. If I went into a certain mall entrance, for example, she would have been there waiting. Even if I did not return for three days, she would be there waiting.

Anyways, after the cabin, we moved into a nice house, which was a front and back (rather than a side by side) duplex. The house was owned by a fellow named Stanley, and it was the first time in my life, that I had befriended my landlord. The only drawback on our side of the house was that there was not enough light, the kitchen was a separate entity (which I hate) and there was again, only one bedroom. But the price was right, and I was still trying to save. And so, life on Dirksen began.

# Chapter 10 – Life on Dirksen

The location was great…it was close to the main part of town, and all the stores. We liked living there, although we had some strange things happening, like our firewood getting stolen. One day a friend of mine had gone out to get some wood, and sure enough, found an extra hand in the woodpile. At the end of the hand was my neighbour who lived in the other side of the house. The worst part was when my sister in law, kookoo Wanda came over, and we went next door for an invited drink. She ended up with Fred, and the trouble really began. They did a lot of crack together, and I made the fatal error of doing it with them a couple of times.

One night, or shall I say, rather, one morning, after doing the shit all night long, Wanda finally left to go over to Fred's. We had run out. It was about 5 am, and I had just crawled into bed wondering how the hell I was ever going to get to sleep. The next thing I know, she was knocking on the door. I thought if I ignored her long enough she would eventually go away. No, not happening, the window was next. I tried to ignore that too, and the next thing I heard was Wanda shouting through the windows and doors. She kept telling me that she had left a "rock" in the bathroom, and that I must let her in to find it. "Jeez," I thought, "that's all I need, is for the neighbours to hear this." Needless to say, I let her back in, and watched sadly as she searched my bathroom floor on her hands and knees, coming up empty handed, of course.

My nearest neighbours had about as many parties and after the bar visitors as I did, and we all hung with the same crowd. One I will always remember though is the party that I threw on behalf of my friend Kathy's birthday party. Kathy did not use coke, and asked that I make sure no one brought it to "her" party. Big mistake, I learned then and there, that you should never tell people not to bring drugs to your party. There was more there than usual. Oh, yes, I forgot to mention. Things had changed by now, no one had to go to Nanaimo anymore, since there were now five big dealers on the island. All you had to do was call, and they would deliver, 24/7.

And, of course , after a few "no thank you's," I caved, and ended up in the bathroom with someone who had invited me in for some lines. I almost shit myself when I heard Kaytlin out in the hallway. The next thing I knew, she was knocking on the door, demanding to know what we were doing in there. I had completely forgotten that Kaytlin and her best friend Ann were home that night. I will never forget coming out of the bathroom, and trying my best to avoid her. The coke had sobered me right up. Now I was really feeling paranoid. I went to quietly sit on the couch, and when I looked over, Kaytlin and Ann were both staring at me. I have never in my life been more uncomfortable. I just could not handle it, and I was sure that they knew what was going on in the bathroom. So, when Teresa, then my neighbour in the back, (Fred had been kicked out, because he couldn't make his rent), suggested that she and I and two guy friends take a drive up to her place to go "smoke some." I was in. I asked Kathy to watch the girls, while I went out for a quick drive.

When we got to Teresa's, we cooked up what we had left, and proceeded to smoke it. I ended up tweaking so badly, and being so scared to go back and face my kid, that they ended up leaving me there all alone. They could not convince me to leave, when they had run out. They did not want to wait for me to "come down." "We'll come back and get you," they lied, and off they took, to go back to the party. I ended up stuck there all night, there was no way to get a hold of them, and they weren't answering the phone at my house. Probably didn't even hear it ring.

Well...the next morning was Mother's Day, which I had also completely forgotten about. Until the phone rang in Teresa's bedroom where I had finally fallen asleep, and it was her mother. I was so stunned by her call, that I had no answer to give her as to where Teresa was, and ended up telling her that she would have to ask Teresa herself. It wasn't until about 11 am that someone finally showed up and took me back to my place. It was about noon by now, and there were Kathy, Kaytlin, and Ann, sitting at the dining room table eating vegetable beef soup. See, the strange things we recall? I recall what soup they were eating! Some guy was still passed out on my living room floor. Never, in my life, had I ever felt like such a shitty mother, ever. Never had I ever, allowed Kaytlin to see me all messed up before. It was awful, and I really didn't know what to say. I simply apologized for fucking up.

And so, another day and another party had transpired on Gabriola Island. Then we heard that Teresa was moving out, because she and Stanley, the landlord had also come to some sort of disagreement. Stan, who had entered our lives, and came around quite a bit now, suggested that Kaytlin and I move into the other side of the house. The back side looked out over a really nice lawn, and then down a bit of an incline with a huge forest behind it, as far as the eye could see. It was a two story, three bedroom upstairs. It had a gorgeous Jacuzzi tub with marble staircase, set in a corner window overlooking the yard in the bathroom. Downstairs was a massive living/dining room, and open concept kitchen. There were lots of windows and so much light. The rent was only a couple of hundred dollars more per month, because he really wanted us in there.

It was Kaytlin though, that talked me into it. "We have always moved, mommy," she said, "and I am bored and need to move again. I admit it," she stated, "I'm addicted to moving." It was so cute, and so with further ado, I made the decision to move for Kaytlin. This left the back suite open, and my really good friends, Chastity and her boyfriend took it. They were the best neighbours anyone could ask for. Lou was out of town working a lot, and so Chas and I began hanging out more and more together. Chastity was good to hang out with, because she didn't do drugs, she didn't even drink. Strange, since she was an entertainer and singer, and she still went to the bars and parties. She always seemed more comfortable to be there whenever I was with her. Others often made her feel guilty for NOT doing drugs.

Stan started coming around more and more, and was often invited to join our dinner table. He had recently gotten a divorce, and I knew that he was lonely. He had two young children, whom he also had over once in a while. It seemed as though all of the single women on the island were in love with Stanley, but he was not able to make it work with anyone. I assumed he wasn't ready. I gather that he was trying to save some money, and his wife had moved to Nanaimo, and that cost him a lot. He asked if I would mind if he put his trailer in the back yard and stay there once in a while. I had no objection, even though "once in a while" turned into a permanent residence. I would allow him to come in and use the shower whenever he needed, and I had no problem with that either. In return he paid for my hydro bill, which was quite steep in the winter. It was a big place to heat, and he had not built it very well.

I no longer worked now in Nanaimo for the call centre. The company had the best benefits package in the city. Rather than allow it to kick in after three months work, they would release the employees, and then ask that they reapply. In my case, it was exactly three months to the very day. Three supervisors called me into a fish bowl of an office, to tell me that they had a tape where I was rude to a customer, and therefore had to let me go. Why it took three people to come up with that, I will never know, other than that they probably knew that I would not take this well. I had seen it coming, and I was very verbal. Everyone there knew me. Long story short, I did not want this to happen to any more people, it was complete dirty play. It would have bothered me forever, had I not fought the claim, and in fact won, hands down. I was able to prove quite easily really, that they had taken a recording, and misconstrued it. They used only a portion of the actual tape, and threw it completely out of context. In reality, I had been joking with the client.

The next job I landed, (and of course I still had my taxes and accounting business, which had grown over time) was at the Twin Beaches grocery store. It was fun working there. It was a little corner store, with a movie rental business, and just about everyone on the island came through there at one point or another. I found that in the new part of the house, my drug use and party mode once again increased in intensity. I had more privacy there, away from Kaytlin, since her bedroom was now upstairs. Were she to get up, I would hear her in time to ditch the evidence.

Now, it is time to tell you another story about the second time that I almost overdosed. I had begun hanging out with a woman that used to waitress at the bar. You would never have guessed that she was a crack head, but Josie was really hardcore. She was a single mother with two small children, whom I felt sorry for. Josie rented a house right on the beach. It was such a beautiful setting. The first time I was there, I had been invited to a house party. By all appearances, such as in my own case, no one would have guessed any of it. I knew that Josie used me a lot to buy the stuff, but I didn't care, it was somehow better than using alone. She had a big rambling house, and there were so many sounds, that I would usually hide out in her bedroom. I wonder still what her kids must have thought. She was usually in and out whenever they were home, trying to keep them occupied. Mostly though, I just went over there when the father had the children, because it made me feel guilty to use around them.

I would sit in her room, and do a big hit, and then sit on her bed and tweak, making sure all the curtains were closed, so no one could see me. When the kids weren't home, we would use downstairs, usually at the dining table. Now, the thing with Josie was that, she did more than I was used to doing, and so not to be left in the dust, (and all out of my money) I also did more. We considered that we were having fun, waiting for the next hoot, while playing cards or dice or something. I began going out less and less. Whenever I did go by the bar now, I was usually in and out, just there to score. My friends began to catch on, and voiced their concerns, but to no avail.

With the sounds of the surf, came a lot of apparitions for me. It became an obsession almost, that I anticipated my brother and my parents were going to sneak up in the back of the house, and be able to see us through the windows, and I would be caught. Sometimes, I made Josie hang blankets or sheets over the windows, just to appease me. One evening, as she sat with her back to the dining room window, I actually saw my brother peering in, behind her. Of course, when I voiced it, she did not see the same thing, telling me that there was no one there.

Well, there was one night in particular, when we had been going all day (a gorgeous sunny summer day as I recall), and it was well into the night, perhaps near morning. We had been out several times to get more, and also had the dealers deliver. I have no idea how much we had consumed, but it happened again. I will always have these images burnt into my memory banks, more real than real actually is. I had done a couple of big hits, right by the stove where we had cooked it. I was melted into the floor, just in front of the stove. I remember loading my pipe with shaking fingers, again hoping that I would not get caught. The ocean waves were rushing in my head already, as I proceeded to light the pipe.

Oh, those familiar snap, crackle, pop sounds, of the cocaine melting into the screen, as the sweet smoke filled my lungs. I knew it was a good hit, for most of them are a letdown after so many hours of use. The next thing I know, I was shaking on the floor like a leaf, uncontrollably. I tried to close my eyes, but I could not, because I knew beyond a shadow of a doubt that my dad was watching with horror through the kitchen window. I felt him, and the next thing I knew, there seemed to be a time lapse, from when he must have climbed through the window to the moment that he stood, looming straight before me. He just stood there looking down on me with sadness and pity. This made me shake even harder, and I honestly thought that I was going under. As I held out a shaking hand to touch him, which was the bravest thing that I could think of to do, he slowly vanished, right before my very eyes.

Again, it seemed, I had beat the odds, and had been so damned close to an overdose, that I thought my heart would stop. Just like when I saw Kaytlin at the end of my bed, this incident was more real to me than almost anything. I believe to this day, Kaytlin and my father, (in both instances) must have been thinking about me, and somehow ended up on another time line to reach out and save me. I honestly, to this day, think that had they not been there, I would have died. You would not be reading this book now. It is so very hard to explain these "out of body" experiences, to people that have never even tried drugs. That day scared me straight for a week or so, and that was a long time, this particular summer. This would have been the summer of 2004, to be precise.

Now, let's get back to the house and my landlord, for it became quite the predicament by year end. Stan was a lonely man, and began coming over more and more. He had gone out with a singer/performer named Claudette, who was truly in love with him, but it didn't work out either. One evening, we were all invited to this party at an old haunted restaurant, that a couple had bought and had just completed renovations in. Stan and I ended up going there together, in my car. I got this weird feeling all of a sudden that he perhaps thought this was a date. When he looked at me lovingly, and planted a big kiss on me, (that I was totally unprepared for) I knew I had to get out of there quickly. It just felt so uncomfortable.

It was shortly after that night, that he came by one afternoon, to take a shower. I was sitting downstairs in the living room, watching television. A while later, he came downstairs, wearing only a towel covering him from the waist down. Before I knew what happened, he stood before me in the dining room, and without further ado, he suddenly dropped his towel. Flabbergasted, I said, "What are you doing?" He wasn't sure what to do then, and turned around pointing at his butt, and said, "Oh, I just wanted you to have a look at this thing. What you think it is?" At quick glance it looked like a mole to me, and not knowing what to do, I said, "Stan, I think you should put your towel back on, and get out of here." It was a most awkward situation. Poor guy turned beet red. And, it was after that, that things began to really go sideways.

It was coming up to the end of 2004, and I had since lost my job at the corner store. The island is small and a new ass hole had arrived. It was because of her, tattling on me about something to do with the video rentals, that my manager showed up at my door to ask me not to return. I had no fight left in me, so I let it go. This woman was one of those toxic people who would have just escalated matters further. Long and short of it is that I was once again broke. I had a few accounting clients, but not enough to pay the bills. Barely enough to buy the drugs.

November arrived and we were in the throes of a Gabriola winter wonderland. We had about two to three feet of snow that year. When I was late on the rent for the first time, Stanley became a different person. Maybe it had something to do with the fact that I was no longer inviting him over as readily. He stayed in his trailer more since the dining room ordeal. Anyway, he decided that cutting my power in the middle of winter was a good idea, and that is exactly what he did. Kaytlin and I were not able to sleep upstairs now. Being that I always find a way to make due, I ran an extension cord into the utility room, and hooked up a base heater, my TV, and a hot plate and coffee pot. I had to keep it all in the living room, where it would reach. Before I knew it, Stanley "broke in," for he did not have permission. He let himself into Lou and Chastity's suite, when they were at work, and cut off the entire power in the house right from the main power box.

I was still able to keep the downstairs warm with my wood stove, but Chas's stove pipes were plugged. They had to suffer even more, because Stan had cut their wires by accident as well. I mean he cut the wires, the actual wires, in his rage. Apparently now, he wanted the rent and the hydro paid for at once. It was only a week into November, when he got his rent money. December 1st arrived, and Stan was back at the door. I saw the look of pure amazement when I pulled out $650 cash, and gave it to him. He told me he wanted me out, and I told him that when I could afford to move, I would. I'm not sure what provoked him next, but there was an island wide power outage after another big snowstorm. My friend Josie and her two kids came over to stay a couple of nights. All of her water pipes had frozen and one had burst at her place on the beach. My brother was on the island working at the time, and he was staying with us also. He had a camper van in the driveway, where he slept.

I don't know if Stan thought that perhaps we hadn't suffered enough. The next thing we knew, we heard some commotion outside. We all looked out to see the city snow plough in my driveway. Stan worked for the island works yard, up keeping the roads. He had brought over the city equipment and proceeded to put two huge mountains of snow behind all of our vehicles, blocking us all into the driveway. There was no other way out! So, there we were stuck for another two days. My brother's hoses in his camper froze and blew. He had been plugged into the house when the power had been cut.

I ran out of wood to heat the place, but luckily, Stan had built a nifty little fence using raw wood. We used the fence, what else was a girl to do? Stan had blocked us in on the weekend, so we were not able to get a hold of the works yard. Monday morning I called, and told them what their idiot employee had done. They made him come and undo the snow piles, or deal with the cops. Now, I forgot, that he had done this another time before. He was mad at me about something, but he had come in with the works plough, and proceeded in dumping a load of gravel right behind my car. What a nut bar!

January 1st came around and by now he had taken me to the tenancy branch with a legal eviction notice. The bastard used the hydro bills, which he had told me not to worry about, and said that I owed him the back pay. I was not able to prove otherwise, and so by January's end, I knew I had to leave. How could one stay after all that anyways? But, what the hell was I to do? I made a decision, and it was mostly due to Kaytlin's age, that I decided to move off the island. Shitty thing was, though, that the little Rabbit Volkswagen I now owned, blew it's engine, and ended up stuck in Josie's driveway. I was now without a vehicle to get off the island in.

Oh, yes, the Daytona. I had been over on the mainland to go to my friend Laura's wedding, and on the way back to the ferry, the engine seized in my Daytona. What was so strange about that, is that it was in exactly the same spot that my brother's engine had also seized in one of his vehicles. The exact same spot! What are the odds? Kaytlin was now in grade eight, and she was fourteen years old. After grade 7, elementary school, the kids go to Nanaimo to attend high school. Now she had to take the ferry every day. I had no car, so she had to try to get rides, or once in a while, she even had to walk all the way. It sucked. Also, at that age, the kids on Gabriola begin "partying," and the 20 something year old boys start picking up the young girls. I had seen it time and again, and I was damned if that was going to happen to my daughter.

I was lucky enough to befriend a fellow by the name of Chris, a super nice guy, and he loaned me $1000 to purchase a car, so that I could make the move. It ended up being one of the toughest moves I had ever endured. I had to move, there was no question, but I had no where to go. There were no rentals available in Nanaimo at this time, that I could afford. I had no choice but to acquire a storage unit to put our belongings into. I boxed up everything at the house, and since Stanley wanted it right out, I put everything in the back overhang. I took what I could over in my car, and hired a truck to take the large load. There were no big hiccoughs until I packed up the water cooler. Stan had purchased it for us when we moved into the first side of the house. We were on a well, and a cistern system there for water, and it was undrinkable. What I didn't realize, is that he thought I would leave it with the house, and if so, all he had to do was ask.

Then the unthinkable happened. While I was out, Stan must have let himself in, again. Everything that was in my office, was gone. I had been so proud that I had everything backed up onto disks, but the son of a bitch took those too. My computer, printer, fax machine, all of my files, and all my backup disks, everything, was gone. Now, aside from the fact that in February it is tax season in Canada, and my busiest time of the year, I soon realized that all the personal records of all my clients past and present were now compromised. What a nightmare I now found myself in. I had no money, and the job that would have seen us through, was now gone. Of course, at this point, I still had hope that he would return everything. But I soon found out that that was not going to happen.

Stan, of course claimed to know nothing about it. Since there was no sign of forced entry, I had no case, right?

About a month prior to that, I had had to call the cops, when Stan showed up at my door, angry as hell about something. I pretended that I was not home, and sat silently on the staircase, as I heard him trying to break in. See, usually, he let himself into the other suite when Lou and Chas were not home, and broke into my place from there. There was a closet and then a laundry room that connected the two suites. He must not have had the key with him that day. When I realized that he was not leaving, I called the cops. Now, on Gabriola Island, when you call them, you actually call Nanaimo, who then dispatches the Gabe officers. I also discovered that when there is a power outage on the island, you cannot reach the cop shop at all, because their answering machine is then not working! Yup, that is right, what a system.

I had a female police officer on the phone, and was giving her a play by play as to what was happening, when I heard a key in the door, and my heart almost stopped. I peeked down the stairwell, and slowly slunk down, the cop still on the phone. As I reached the bottom of the stairs, I saw Kaytlin come through the doorway, and Stan trying to push in right behind her. "Please stay outside," I asked him. Then I proceeded to hand him the phone, saying, "Here, this call is for you." He sure did look surprised when he discovered he was talking to the police. They told him to leave the property, and thankfully, he did.

And so, when I realized that he had no intention of returning my property, (the computer was brand new by the way) I called the police to report the incident. They told me that they would stop by and have a word with him, but that beyond that, there would not be anything they could do. They had no idea where he would have put the computer. "It could be at the bottom of the ocean, for all we know," they told me. When the cops did show up to talk to Stan, he told them that he thought that my brother Matt had stolen my things, and gave the cops his address, and sent them to his door.

So, let's get to when we actually found ourselves on the other side of the water, and in Nanaimo, with no where to go. I did not know what to do, I had never been in this much of a pickle in my life. I had a kid and a dog, and no place to lay our heads. And so, I found us a cheap motel. All I could afford was a single room, a tiny one, with two single beds and a small bathroom. We had to sneak Sally in! And so, we grabbed a few clothes, and our toiletries, and ended up living there for a good month, while I tried to find us another place.

My mother and father in law lent us a coffee maker. I blew it up trying to use it as a hot plate to warm up soup. Next, I purchased a little hot plate to heat things up, and the dishes had to be done in the bathroom sink or the bathtub. It was a sad state of affairs, and I cannot recall ever feeling like more of a loser than I did at this low point in my long life. I could not even provide for my little family. For all I had been through before this, I did not deserve this, that much I knew. But I suppose there is a reason for everything, and if it doesn't kill you...well, you know, we keep hearing that.

My girlfriend Kathleen had also moved from Gabriola Island, and it was a beautiful sunny day. Kaytlin had gone to school, and was staying with the grandparents, or a friend that night. I went to pick up Kathleen, and we ended up at the rowdiest bar in Nanaimo. I met this fellow there, and he invited me to go out for a hoot. I had never done this before, but I was already pretty wasted, and so I wasn't thinking or caring rationally. We went to my car, which was parked on the main drag right in front of the club. Out came the crack pipe, and we smoked it right there. I recall looking out the windows of the car, and seeing all the homeless souls huddled in doorways, doing the same thing I was doing in my car. I felt an odd kinship in that moment. It wasn't long before I began tweaking and worrying about getting caught, especially after Kathleen discovered what we were up to.

And so, I invited this guy back to the motel room. It turned out that he was a dealer, and he had loads of the shit. I tried to keep up to him, but it was impossible. Kathleen looked scared and disgusted, so I tried not to look at her too much. After I thought I was going to overdose a couple of times, I finally realized that this was not fair to my friend, who was clearly uncomfortable. I finally asked the guy to leave. I'm not sure, but he must have left me a couple of hoots. The next thing I know, I was lying on the bed, feeling as though I was overdosing...that shaky horrible feeling, when you try to hang on to life. I was shaking like a leaf, and I know it was scaring poor Kathleen. When I finally stopped with the shaking, and Kathleen knew I was okay, it had hit daybreak. That was when she took off out of there, saying that she would take a bus back. I still feel so bad for putting her through this, and told her so on a recent visit.

I must have fallen asleep, and it was after noon when I woke back up. I knew that I had once again come near death, a third time lucky. I lay there wondering why I was doing these horrible things to myself, and how it affected Kaytlin. I hated Nanaimo already. I had the same feelings of oppression when we came through Nanaimo when I was young. It is an old city, that is dilapidated, and poor, and full of drugs and crime. It feels when you wander through, as though everyone is tweaking at their windows. I will never forget the evening that a friend from Gabe took me out for dinner and dancing. It was a balmy summer evening, on a Saturday night. As we walked down the deserted sidewalks at like 8 pm, there were no cars and no people to be seen. I could not help feeling as though we were in a deserted ghost town, with zombie-like creatures laying in wait. I clutched my purse a little tighter. It made no sense to us, when I brought up the topic. Yes, Nanaimo was the most depressed, oppressed city that I had ever resided in.

So, the next place that I found through a friend of mine, was in a tidy little two storey house, that would entail living with a roommate. Darnell, the fellow who lived there, was a roofer who worked with my friend Tia. It ended up being the strangest living arrangement, and was never comfortable for myself or for Kaytlin. She and I had to share a room, and Darnell was away at work on weekdays. When he came home, he would disappear into his room and hang out in there all the time. It didn't take a rocket scientist to figure out that he was getting high in there a lot.

The laundry was shared with a young woman who lived downstairs with her kid. She was a total crack head. There would be people coming in and out all day and all night long. My clothes started to go missing out of the laundry room. She tried to come upstairs all the time, for one thing or another, and I had to shut it down from the start. I had to tell her that I did not have the time to answer the door, or wait for her to make her calls, or watch her kid. This did not create a loving relationship between us, and caused even more clothes to go missing, and an underlying animosity towards me, but I had my own problems. All in all we did not feel safe.

We lasted there about two months before we could not take the oppressed feelings anymore, and I decided to move back to Vancouver, whatever it took. I packed up my stuff, got ripped off for my damage deposit and another half a month's rent. Since there was only about a month or so left of school, I took a shot in the dark, and asked my mom to keep Kaytlin until the end of the school year. I had no money to hire a truck this time. Don't forget, I could not do my taxes.

What I did forget to mention however, was that before I moved, I had once again taken my real estate course. I had received a call one evening from my "angel on earth," and Georgia told me that I had to take the course again. She would loan me the money, if I agreed. The course was so dry and boring the second time through. I did what I call "commercial studying," at the same time smoking a ton of weed so that I would not want to go out. The course consists of five different kinds of law, and mortgage brokerage. Nothing in those books teaches us how to sell a house, believe me. It is all about how to cover your ass legally.

I had tried to find work in Nanaimo, but things were really bad at that time, and no one was hiring. The office I tried to get into as a Realtor, made me feel like a total loser, when they discovered that I had no money. I had already been accepted, and had foolishly brought in my new "lucky" trinkets to put on my new desk. I was so chagrined by the entire experience, that I did not go back to pick up my belongings.

So, I left KK at my mom's, who had just stepped up to the plate for the first time in my life. I loaded up the car with what I needed most, and took off back to Vancouver. There, I stayed with my best friend from high school, (Mandy) and her boyfriend, in an apartment, close to town. As I began the job quest, I stumbled upon a position for a receptionist in a real estate office. Real estate is a self employment field of business, guys, that requires about $20,000 to enter comfortably. When I went for the interview however, the two fellows who owned the office, convinced me to start right away, as a realtor (not receptionist). They made extravagant promises to help me get on my feet, and so I bit.

It was a prestigious office in location only. The office was right at the entrance to Library Square on Robson Street in Vancouver, BC. It is considered to be one of the city's prime locations. What I did not take into consideration, amongst so many other things, was the price it would cost to park everyday. Whenever you had to go to another office, like city hall for instance, it would cost again, and again. If I could only describe to you all in words just how much of a struggle I was going through.

I had my dog, who could not stay in the apartment. Sally had to stay in my car. I would have to go out and check on her often. Oh, yes, and now I remember that there was a back window missing in my car, which Stanley had also broken in anger. One late afternoon, I went out to take Sally for a walk, and she was gone. The whole thing was such a nightmare, that it did not seem real. I barely had time to miss my daughter, and was just grateful that she did not have to endure this with me. Again guys, I had no idea how hard it would be to write this book. I hate having to relive these dark days. Let us not forget that I was also kicking the crack at this time, and when the chips are down, an addict wants it even more.

My mom struggled with Kaytlin, who was not as neat and tidy as we were moulded to be. She sent her over to her other grandma's, (now in Nanaimo) whenever she could. I tried to get on my feet as quickly as possible. Having taken on the realtor role without money had been a stupid move, and no one helped me as promised. I got a deal within a week of getting into the office, and my licence had not even come through yet. Now, what was I to do? Well, I looked around, and picked the hungriest person in the office, another new struggling realtor. I figured that someone new could use the commission more than a seasoned person. And so Heather and I co-listed a condo very far away in a neighbouring town called Langley. As luck would have it, my license came in a week after the sale, and commission split!

Long story short once again, we sold the unit one day before the listing was supposed to have expired. The partner I chose ended up with my client, which is not ethical in any business. There went my repeat customer. So, half of the commission, (and it still gives me goose bumps) added up to exactly $1,111 after all was said and done. I may well have forgotten to tell you all, that since Gray's death, the number 11:11 presented itself so often, that it simply could not be ignored. It began coming up more and more now. All of my good friends and family know about it, and what 11:11 means to me. That is why, since I am nearly done writing, I plan to publish this book on 11:11:11!

It happened after Kaytlin joined me in Vancouver. All of our coats and shoes were in the trunk, when it happened. Kaytlin was safe at Auntie Mandy's apartment, and I had reconnected with Cory (the realtor with the boat). Corey and I ended up going out to his boat for a few drinks. It was when I left later on that night, that I was pulling out of the marina and onto Barnett Highway, that it happened. It was one of those moments in time that one cannot explain. True, I should not have been drinking and driving, but where I had come from and what I had done, drinking and driving was not unheard of. It used to be that if a cop pulled you over, and you were plastered, they would ask how much farther you had to go. If someone else was in the car, they would allow them to drive, or they would tell you to be careful. It used to be so easy to get away with so much back in the day. However, this night, the drinking was not a factor in my tale.

As I pulled through the parking lot, I ran across a guy who waved me over. His buddies' boat had broken down, and he was left to his own devices to get home. He explained in the car, that he was going in the opposite direction from me, or I would have given him a ride home. I pulled up to the stop sign, at the exit of the marina, and let the gentleman out of my car. Now, bear in mind, that I am in a stationary position at this time. I nudged my car out and looked both ways. There was not one vehicle on the highway, in either direction.

I took another look right, and then left, as I turned left onto the road. Out of nowhere, I caught the bright red colour of motion, and it was bearing directly down on me. There was no time to react, I thought, "this is it," and then the impact. The other vehicle hit my tail end on the driver's side. I jumped out of the car and ran over to see if they were okay. Sitting, looking pretty shaken up was an older couple. All they both said was that they had not seen my big white car at all. I told them that I had not seen their bright red car at all either. Yet, we had collided. I still cannot explain where that car had come from, and I know, neither can they.

At this point I do not recall how I got home, whether I called Corey, and he took me home, or what? My car, however, ended up in the impound yard, and I did not afford to get it out. So, there it sat for a few days collecting charges, and it was then I called Ralph to help me. He lent me the money and we called to pick it up. They tow yard told me that they had buried the car in the back of their lot, and needed another day to get it out. So, the next day, Ralph picked me up, and we went down to the yard. They still had the car buried, and so we waited, until they brought it out to the front of the shop. Everything had been stolen out of the trunk (which now would not close) and so KK and I were left without any shoes, boots, and coats. A few kitchen items remained. Here's the weird part. By the time, Ralph and I paid the charges and walked out to the car, someone had stolen the license plate, right there in broad daylight! So, now I had to go and pay for another plate, and of course had to borrow even more money.

Now it was KK and I, (with poor Sally in the car) staying at Mandy's apartment. I knew that it would only last so long, and began saving like crazy. I spent another $2000, from my second commission, to buy another car. This car had been primed to paint, and would have looked good, had I ever gotten that far. But again, things got messed up, can you imagine? I had just found some new clients a home to buy, and it was their moving day. My mother was in town, and I brought her with me, to bring the young couple a bottle of champagne. My new car was parked right in front of the house on the road. We were there for maybe 45 minutes, before we decided to leave. I could not believe my eyes when I saw that my new car was all smashed up in the back. It was a hit and run, right there, just like that.

There was nothing I could do, since I had no collision. I had not been able to afford it, and didn't think I would need it. My whole life, I had always put collision on my vehicles, except for this one particular instance. Surprise? Not at all. Oh, wait, let me rephrase that. There was one other time, when I bought a total shit box. I had always paid cash for my cars in the past. I had purchased a total beater, and therefore, I thought, no one would even think to steal it. "Who cares if it gets damaged?" I had thought. Well... it got stolen, tires taken off, sunroof taken out, all the papers missing. Yup, Petra luck!

Mandy's apartment did not last very long. There was too much pressure on everyone, and after a huge blowout with things said that should not have been said out loud, between Mandy and I. I gathered KK and we ended up back on the doorstep of Carmen Lake. No matter what, I have always been able to count on her, and value her friendship so much. It was not long after we started staying there, that we finally lost our poor Silly Sally. Sally had had to stay on the porch outside, because one of Carmen's boys was allergic to dogs. Sally's only desire has always been just to be by my side, and she was not at all happy with this arrangement. It was Halloween, fireworks went off, and the next thing I knew she was gone. We put up flyers and did all we could, but Sally was never to return. I still think about her everyday, and hope she is in a good place, with people that love her.

After spending a few months at Carmen's, I managed to get KK and I another basement suite. We rented what Kaytlin and I would end up referring to as the blue house. It was a really bright blue, spacious basement suite. This was also about the same time, (and I feel I need to feel you all about it now) that I experienced what I now call "the last hurrah." One day, there was a knock on the door, and before me stood a young girl, whom I knew I recognized. It turned out to be my cousin Heidi's daughter, a couple years younger than my own. She had heard that we lived there, and it was not far from my cousin's place. I gave her a ride home, and before long, my cousin and I began hanging out. The shitty thing was that Heidi was a crack head, and before long I caved and began using with her again. I really did not want to start doing it at my place again though, as I had done in the past. I felt so bad, that I had taken another fall.

This went on for about a month or two, and of course, it was usually me buying the stuff. What else was new? Let me jump right ahead though, and tell you about this one night in particular. Heidi lived in a dark suite, just like the ones I hated. Upstairs lived a crossed eyed hooker. Heidi and I had been out together that day, and decided to score on the way home. The hooker came downstairs and we offered her some too. Then we ran out, and I finally caved and bought us all some more. When we had finished that together, the hooker decided to go out and "pull a trick" to get us more. It was well into the night by now, and Heidi and I both decided to lay down while we waited for her to return with the goods.

I dozed off, and awoke when I heard something in Heidi's room. I realized then, that they were hiding in there and probably doing the shit without me. That made me feel so horrible. How could I have allowed all of this crap to happen again? Weren't there always fights and bad feelings surrounding drug use in my past?

I laid back, and for the first time in a long time, I asked for help. I begged Gosh for help. I begged Gosh to please release me from this horrible hold that these horrible drugs had over me. I completely surrendered to Gosh that night.

Suddenly I felt a warmth wash over me, as though someone were holding me in their arms. Before I knew what I was doing, I calmly walked over to Heidi's bedroom door. Without even knocking, I turned the handle, and sure enough, there they were. They sure did look guilty, realizing that I had just caught them. I looked at Heidi, and calmly said, "Heidi, I want you to lose my number, and I do not want to hear from you again." With that I closed the door, got into my car, and drove home and went to bed. That night was the last night, that I ever used the shit again. That was July 2005.

My next step was a plan to buy a new car off the lot, one that would be presentable for work. My friend Georgia, helped me by co-signing for the loan. That is when my real struggle began. I worked like a dog every day. I tried and I tried to make a go of real estate. So often I did not have enough money for gas to take clients out house hunting, but I always managed to find a way. I had this great idea to have a seminar, and I called it "Real Estate for Woman." I found myself three volunteers to help me plan and market it, and I paid for all the ads. I put over $2,000 into it, believing that it would get me more business. I was lucky enough to recruit the Mayor of my town to be our keynote speaker, and a televised mortgage broker, to be the other speaker. It was to be a big affair, at an elite golf course venue.

At the very last moment I had no choice but to back out. There were not enough tickets presold, and everyone said they would get one at the door. Since the catering expense was going to be so large, I did not trust it, and pulled out. Then, I had to come up with the money to pay everyone back, and it had already been spent! Another Petra nightmare, and certainly not for lack of trying. During one of our evening volunteer meetings, I had dropped my laptop to help one of my volunteers with something. Soon after that, my computer crashed, causing even more "business problems." I lost all of my contacts and work documentation. What a pain!

So...first, I lose my first client to that other female realtor. Then, my car gets totalled in a hit and run. I then double ended a listing, which means that I listed the house, and found the buyer. Wow... good stuff! Then I get another listing, and it gets really ugly. It is a divorce situation, and I really needed the money, so long story short, the couple's brother ends up buying it. But not until after Petra the idiot, decreases her own commission by a whopping $7,000, in order to make the deal fly. On the last day of the listing! I have never told anyone about that since. I was so embarrassed to be that desperate. But, I had bills to pay. Every time I got a commission, the office would take it all, because my fees would have accumulated.

Next, along comes this really funny, totally kooky, black woman. She was referred to me by another realtor. I am guessing he knew that she would be trouble. She was a first time home buyer, and so all the finances are scrutinized closely by the bank. She had one last outstanding T4 (wage document) to get in to the bank, having passed all the finance tests. She had already written up the offer, which had been accepted, hinging only on this last bit of paperwork. I had lined up an inspection of the house, and the inspector had already been paid, so why should Petra worry about a thing?

Well...let me tell you again, about the Petra luck. The last wage form she was to get in DID NOT EXIST! She had lied about a third job, knowing that they would turn her down without that income! Yup, the deal fell apart swiftly after that...it only took one embarrassing phone call.

And so, with that, let's talk about the last Petra Hoffmann deal. I finally landed my first million dollar listing, and boy, did it feel good! I was so exuberant. I had no money to market it, but I worked it out and market it I did! I spent a lot of money driving one of the seller's sons around to look for their next home. Pretty hard to say, "No, I can't really afford the gas, now isn't it?" I was pretty happy to get a call or email from Saskatchewan one day, about one month away from the end of that listing. It was from a couple whose kids live in Vancouver, and so they were looking to buy out here, to be closer to their family. I spent weeks, sending them video, pictures, city plans, everything I could find to make sure they were comfortable not only with the house, but also with their new neighbourhood. We lined up a date for them to come out to see the house in person and make the offer. Then I got the Petra call. The woman in question had just sustained a heart attack, and all their plans would have to be put on hold. Yup...that couple is still in Saskatchewan, now struggling terribly, for Gay's health did not and has not gotten any better.

For a moment now, I am going to take you back to the Island. I knew in my heart that my father had fallen in love with his new "business partner." I felt sorry for my little brother. Matt has worked with my dad his entire life, has given everything of himself. Without a word to anyone my dad had him removed from all the signage, as well as from the business cards. There was no apparent reason, other than perhaps "She" had wanted it that way. "She," who in the long run, ended up stealing his business right out from under him.

Now, rather than have the balls to tell my mom that he was leaving her, he just slowly began moving his belongings over to the cabin. Feigning business, he started to stay there more and more, having "She" also coming back and forth from the mainland now. This all transpired after 44 years of marriage. I suppose that my parents were both surprised that I had left the island. My mother still blames me for the fact that she is stuck on Gabriola by herself. She truly in her heart seems to believe that it is fully my fault.

So, now while I was struggling to make a go of real estate, and things were finally starting to pick up for me, I received a terrible call from Vancouver Island. My mom was in the hospital, having flat lined twice, a couple of days prior to the call. Apparently, (and to no surprise of my own) I was not listed on any of mom's paperwork. My parents have never told people that I or KK even exist. I went to the island just as quickly as the transportation systems would take me. My mom, had had a cervical biopsy at the hospital. They had cut too deep, which caused her to bleed out into her stomach. The nurses had been about to send her home, when she collapsed. She was rushed into emergency surgery, and died twice on the table.

By the time I got to the hospital, and walked into her room, I did not recognize my own mother. My brother was there, and my dad was on his way. I stayed by my mother's side, and spoke on her behalf with the doctors, nurses and surgeons. My dad and brother wandered in and out, going to Costco to shop together, and stuff, so it was left up to me essentially. I'm sure they will not agree that is how it all happened, but regardless. My family, I realize now, for the first time in my life, is so used to lying about everything, and who and what they are, that they do not even realize it anymore. They even lie to themselves.

I stayed with my good friend Mallory, right by the ferry terminal on Gabriola, for my mom was in Nanaimo hospital. I paid for parking in the city, I paid for all the ferry trips, I paid for all the gas to and from the hospital. This was money I could ill afford. I was there for my mom in every way, but I was not allowed to stay at either her house, or at dad's cabin. My brother stayed at my mom's house, and she even gave him her car keys. See, my parents still do not trust me, they have it in their heads that I will have a giant party in their home or something. They just don't trust me, I have been a drug addict, and that is all they will ever see. They may never see me for who I have become.

I lost two business deals at home, but I felt like I had to stay by her side. To me $12,000 was a small price to pay to be with my family. About two and a half weeks later, after my mom had recovered somewhat in the hospital, she sent me home. She told me, "Thanks, but I don't need you here, I have your brother, who will stay until I get back on my feet." I was astounded, but said nothing. I had no money left to get back to the mainland, and my mother had to give me the money to get back home. She still hangs that over my head.

So...that my friends, was the real thanks I got. I still shake my head over it. My tears have run dry. One good thing did come of it though. As I stood down by the water, waiting for the last ferry to arrive, I was suddenly engulfed by a feeling I had never experienced before. And then it dawned on me. I realized for the first time in my life, that I was home. Gabriola Island was MY home. Having been born in Germany, and having moved around so many times, this feeling was completely foreign to me. It has stuck with me ever since that moment.

Now, let me lay out for you the struggles which I endured with my second attempt at the real estate career. When I got back from the island, it seemed, I was not able to catch up on all of the failures, and losses. The next thing I knew, Kaytlin and I sat in an apartment, for which I could no longer pay the rent. Since my car had been co-signed, there was no way that I could default or let it go. It then became a choice, the apartment or the car. Office fees at my company had eaten up all my income, and now I was getting deeper and deeper in the hole. I was left with no other recourse, (and although I had promised my self years and years earlier that I would never again ask my parents for help) I bit the bullet and made the call. I did not want to put Kaytlin through this again, especially since she had finally found a school she liked. I simply could not move her again. So, with a dread in my heart, I courageously picked up the phone, and dialled my mother's number.

It was one of the hardest things I ever had to do, but I did it. I asked my mom if she could please help us out with one month's rent ($750), so that we did not have to lose our home. She turned me down, point blank. If it had been with the truth, it would not have hurt so much. But when a woman's house is clear title, and that same woman is off on trips all the time, and she says that she cannot do it financially...wow.

Oh, and here is another thing I forgot to tell you about. A few months prior to this, my mom started talking about listing her house on Gabriola Island, so that she could move back to the city, and be amongst her friends. She was all alone on Gabe, and I totally agreed that was the best thing she could do for herself, especially after the hospitalization. But, (and yes, believe it) she would not list the house with me. I then explained to her that she could pick an island realtor, and I could co list it. I explained that if it sold I would get a portion of the commission for the "referral." It is a regular real estate practise. What would it matter to her, other than her own daughter and grandchild receiving some monies out of it, if her house sold? No, she wouldn't do it. My own mother!

And so, we lost the apartment, and found ourselves homeless once again. Not only did I lose the apartment, but I had nowhere to store our newly acquired furniture and belongings, and no money to move it. So, Kaytlin and I took our clothes and bathroom necessities, and left the rest behind. I then called management and told them they could auction it off, or perhaps rent out the unit as a fully furnished apartment. I had a nice living room set, dining room set, and two bedroom suites, everything was left behind.

The worst part of it all was though, was that Kaytlin and I would not be able to be together. There was not enough room at anyone's homes where we could both stay. I cannot tell you guys enough, how much I felt like such a big loser, now more than ever. It was all completely out of my hands and in Gosh's hands now. There was nothing more that I could do. I ended up staying with my brother and his wife, in their crammed apartment. They were both chain-smokers, and everything I owned took on the smell of stale cigarette smoke. I can still smell it. Kaytlin, stayed with her aunt and uncle and cousins.

And so, always having found a way before, I took a job in an office. Again, my angel Georgia had come to my rescue, and offered me the position in her firm. Again, it helped me get back to renting a place for Kaytlin and myself. I took it because it was near KK's school, and my little one had also managed to find a job of her own. It was at a Dairy Queen restaurant and it was only about three blocks away, so she was able to walk to and fro. The suite was so depressing though, because it was in the back of a huge house, partially underground, with a huge cement wall for scenery. I thought I could handle it, but with natural sunlight having always been so important to me, it was dingy and horrid. We pretty much looked at it as a place to change and eat, and to sleep. Kaytlin ended up with her second boyfriend, and stayed at his house a lot. That made it worse for me, because it was really hard to come home on a beautiful sunny afternoon, if she wasn't at least at home.

# Chapter 11 – What is Hepatitis?

Then, as though things were not bad enough, I was about to receive a rather huge blow...it was some time in August 2008, that I had made a doctor's appointment in order to ask him to run some blood work on me. I had been having problems with my stomach, and feeling tired all the time, along with several other symptoms. I had been putting my health off for far too long. It first began when we still lived on Gabriola Island. I started having stomach pains, and could not hold my alcohol. I actually began vomiting whenever I had a drink or two. That was when I first knew that something was wrong inside. I made some appointments at that time, and had some barium tests done. They told me that there was nothing wrong with my stomach, and I took them at their word.

I had been putting off the blood work for at least two years because it is really difficult for me to go in. I have no veins. Having put needles in my arms for years, my veins have completely collapsed. I have found in the past that when you go for blood work, many health care workers do not have a lot of patience for dirty junkies like myself, and it has always been a nightmare. They used the last vein in my hand when I bore Kaytlin. Anyway, this time I had gone, and a few weeks later, I got the call that he wanted to see me.

What transpired next was a total shock, even to me. Although in hindsight, I do not understand why I had not thought of it myself. My doctor had run my blood for everything, since I expressed my concern about my fears of having blood taken. I had specifically asked him to run it for any thyroid and haemoglobin issues, due to my constant fatigue. My doctor of over twenty years standing, told me that day, that I have chronic Hepatitis C. It is a life threatening disease that attacks your liver, and is responsible for most deaths caused by liver disease. I have a lot of friends who have it, and a lot of friends who have died from Hep C.

Deanne was the first person I ever knew that was diagnosed with it, for we knew about Hepatitis A and B, but Hep C had not yet been discovered. The thing I remember the most about Deanne, is that she always complained about being tired all the time. It was tiring to hear it, for she mentioned it almost every day. It turned out years later that Rudy had it too. I do not even know if they are still alive. I have lost track of them. I spoke to Dee last when I went to Vancouver for Fat Cat's funeral. He died of Hepatitis C. She did not want to see me, because she said that she was too sick and looked terrible. She reminded me how vain she was and hoped I would understand, which of course I did.

Alright then, skipping right along as always...I had to wait seven long excruciating months to see the liver specialist to ascertain how much damage my liver had sustained. I don't know if I mentioned earlier, but I had only ever shared a needle once, and it was with Dennis. I was always so careful to use my own, because Rudy and Dee had drilled it into my head, that that is how diseases are transferred between junkies. Hep C is carried only from blood to blood, and although a lot of cases are due to to needles and blood transfusions, Hepatitis C is also contracted from tattoos, piercing, sharing razors, sharing toothbrushes, dental work, etc. Most people that have it, do not tell anyone, because of the huge stigma the disease still carries. It is commonly thought that "only junkies" get Hep C.

Anyway, on April 9th, 2009, I was told that I have "advance chronic liver disease" and most likely cirrhosis of the liver. My specialist reminded me that although I have only known about it for eight months, I have actually had the disease for more than 20 years. That is why they call it the silent killer. By the time most people are diagnosed, the damage has already been done, and more often than not, they are already in end stage liver disease. They call it the silent killer because the liver feels no pain I call it the silent killer because nobody talks about, because they are ashamed and living with the stigma.

We have yet to assess how much damage my liver has sustained, and that will require a liver biopsy. The gastroenterologist wants to put me on the treatment immediately. I am not supposed to have even one drink, but I have been drinking more than I did before the diagnosis. I suppose it goes back to not liking being told what to do. Also, after giving it a weak effort, I realized that the decision will be taken from me once I'm put on the treatment anyways.

I have always thought of myself as being fearless...well maybe not always, but certainly lately. I actually believed that I was afraid of nothing. Now I realize that I was wrong, and really what else is new? I got back home from the liver specialist's office on July 7, 2009. And...for the first time since I have been diagnosed, it is all real to me. I now understand that I am truly sick. I found out only yesterday, that two more people I went to school with have passed away, one of them from Hep C. This has scared me. I now know that I have been in denial up until now. It turns out that Hepatitis C is indeed a life threatening illness. Globally speaking there are 500 million people that have Hepatitis B and C, and 1.5 million die from it each year. I left the doctor's office in a bit of a daze.

Since my initial diagnosis, I have taken it upon myself to research my illness. It turns out that there are many different "strains" of this virus. The two most prevalent in Canada are "genotypes 1 and 2." What I was told now, was that apparently I have genotype 1, and it is the more difficult one to treat. It seems that I would have to be put on the treatment which consists of two different drugs, plus an anti-depressant. I would be put on it for probably one year, not the six months I had initially thought. One of the drugs is called Interferon, which is like a time released chemotherapy. The other is called Ribavirin.

I was also informed at this time that not everyone responds to the treatment. If I were not to respond, (and that is apparently quite common) they will pull me off treatment in three months time. Or, my red cell and white cell count can change so dramatically, that that would present the same outcome. The long and short of it is that I will only have a 45% chance of the treatment even working. That fact on it's own brought me, mentally speaking, to my knees today. I find myself now completely humbled.

After I came back from the specialist's office, I started to think about all I had been told, and how bad it was going to be. I would not be able to work on treatment, I would no longer have a sex life, and then the doctor described how sick I would actually be. The doctor had told me all the things I had been too scared to ask, and it was not pretty at all.

I would lose my hair, my lustre, and my unbelievable zest for life. I began to realize that it would suck the life right out of me. But, before I left Dr Chang's office that day, he mentioned (and I barely heard him at the time) that I may have a choice to put off treatment. Maybe for a year, or too years, depending of course on the many factors of life style, etc. Of course it would also depend on how much damage my liver had sustained. Not having realized that there was a choice at all, I began pondering this as I drove home, and the more I thought about it, the clearer it had already become.

I will share this with you now. I have come to the conclusion, at least for the time being, that I would rather die next week, than to be that sick for a year. Not for a 45% chance of stopping the disease, and more than likely damaging my other organs in the process. I spoke with a friend the other day, who has gone through the same treatment, and it did not work for him. He is dying slowly, and does not look well at all. He is yellow and jaundiced looking. Surprising enough though, he tried to convince me to take the treatment. He said that I may not be that sick at all, and 45% is better than no percent.

I went back to the specialist about a week later, only to talk to him about my decision to refuse treatment. I swear that in my head I was totally good with that decision, thinking that it would be mind over matter. I thought that by refusing treatment, I would simply just be okay. I was later driving from the doctor's office on route to Vancouver General Hospital to visit my uncle, who had just had a lung transplant. I felt as though thoughts were escaping me faster than they were coming to me. They were there and gone again before I could even grasp them.

You see, my doctor had just pulled me out of my warm and cozy bubble, (the one in which I would just be okay after all.) He had received my liver biopsy results, and shared with me that they showed fibrosis and the beginnings of cirrhosis. He pretty much told me that it is really not an option to turn down treatment, and that without it I would certainly die. He insinuated that within two years time, bad things would start to happen to me, if I did not accept treatment. I told my specialist that I had made up my mind, that I simply could not tolerate a whole year of treatment.

I explained that it would strip me of my spirit, and that I would rather die tomorrow than to go through that. I realized that I could not put my family and friends through it with me. I was amazed that he looked so shocked. He told me that he had never heard anyone say that before. I said, "Of course, you must have heard this before, you do this everyday." He then restated that truly, he had never in all his practise heard anyone say anything like that in his experience.

I have since thought it through, and for now I am holding off. I do not wish to be left an empty shell, and that is what I picture. I know what it is like to be sick for six months, and find it unfathomable. Somehow it is all 'so real," and at the same time it is "surreal." It is good enough for me to know that I have finished something. **I have finished this book**. Seriously, the only other thing that I have ever finished in my life was an afghan for my mother! Let us see now, if Gosh lets me write another.

In closing: You must be wondering why I called this book 11 Vials? The number 11:11 first came to me right after Grayson died. Kaytlin and I have seen it ever since. Coming out of the bathroom, and seeing it on three clocks at once, for instance. Everyone close to us sees it now, for they know the story. In my heart and in my soul, I feel as though the number 11:11 is important for all of us somehow.

The reason that I called this book 11 Vials is because that is how many vials of blood were taken from me in the hospital. My specialist had wanted to rule out everything else. It took three nurses, trying to find a big enough vein, to pull that much blood from me that day. When I asked one of them to count the Vials...that was when I knew. The date was April 16, 2009.